An Integrative Approach to Treating Babies and Children

A Multidisciplinary Guide

EDITED BY JOHN WILKS

FOREWORD BY FRANKLYN SILLS

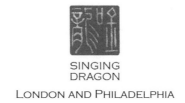

SINGING
DRAGON

LONDON AND PHILADELPHIA

Figure 7.5 amended and reproduced from Ogden *et al.* (2006) with kind permission of Norton.
Figure 7.8 amended and reproduced from Field (1985) with kind permission of Elsevier.

First published in 2017
by Singing Dragon
an imprint of Jessica Kingsley Publishers
73 Collier Street
London N1 9BE, UK
and
400 Market Street, Suite 400
Philadelphia, PA 19106, USA

www.singingdragon.com

Library of Congress Cataloging in Publication Data
Title: An integrative approach to treating babies and children : a
multidisciplinary guide / edited by John Wilks.
Description: London ; Philadelphia : Singing Dragon, 2017.
Identifiers: LCCN 2016042262 | ISBN 9781848192829 (alk. paper)
Subjects: | MESH: Psychology, Child | Infant | Child Welfare | Integrative
Medicine--methods | Psychotherapy--methods | Family Relations--psychology
Classification: LCC RJ504 | NLM WS 105.5.M3 | DDC 618.92/8914-
-dc23 LC record available at https://lccn.loc.gov/2016042262

British Library Cataloguing in Publication Data
A CIP catalogue record for this book is available from the British Library

ISBN 978 1 84819 282 9
eISBN 978 0 85701 229 6

Printed and bound in Great Britain

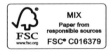

An Integrative Approach to
Treating Babies and Children

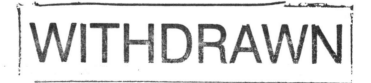

by the same author

Choices in Pregnancy and Childbirth
A Guide to Options for Health Professionals,
Midwives, Holistic Practitioners, and Parents
John Wilks
ISBN 978 1 84819 219 5
eISBN 978 0 85701 167 1

Using the Bowen Technique to Address
Complex and Common Conditions
John Wilks and Isobel Knight
ISBN 978 1 84819 167 9
eISBN 978 0 85701 129 9

DEDICATION

This book is dedicated to babies and children everywhere, who are our greatest teachers and remind us of our deep humanity and connection.

CONTENTS

FOREWORD

Franklyn Sills

I was so pleased to receive the draft of *An Integrative Approach to Treating Babies and Children* from its editor, John Wilks. I have known John over many years and also know a number of the contributors. It is an area of exploration that I have been involved in for a long time, and I am so happy to see the depth and scope shown in this text.

I can remember way back in 1979, my then wife, Maura Sills, returned one evening from a training with Dr William Emerson, one of the pioneers in modern pre- and perinatal psychology. I was not involved in the work at the time. Maura was full of excitement about the workshop and, as we sat in front of the fireplace, she began to share her experiences of the day with William, which involved an exploration of her earliest experiences both in her mother's womb and during her own birth. I sat deeply listening and the next thing I knew, my eyes began to flutter and my body began to move in strange ways. For the next two hours, Maura became my 'midwife', helping me explore my arising birth process. I was actually born two months premature in 1947, which was a dangerous thing at the time, and even today, very challenging. I discovered the little one within me, who was, at his core, still scared, dissociative and disconnected from safety-in-relationship. This event set me off on one of the most important explorations of my life, a reclaiming of my own empowerment 'to be' as I began to access my earliest prenatal and birth processes. William Emerson has become a dear friend and colleague and I have assisted him in many seminars over the last 30 years. Over this time, I helped him clarify some of the concepts that are now part of the work, such as the four stages of the birth process and the importance of mindful inquiry along with appropriate pacing.

At that time, in the 1970s, I was also exploring many humanistic forms of therapy, working deeply with mindfulness practice and exploring various forms of bodywork. This led me into a journey of inquiry and learning, both within the psychotherapy field, where I helped develop one of the world's original mindfulness-based psychotherapy forms, Core Process Psychotherapy and a form of Craniosacral Therapy, known as Craniosacral Biodynamics, which orients to the later work of the founder of Cranial Osteopathy, W. G. Sutherland DO, where the most formative forces of life are at the heart of one's perception. Within this journey Maura Sills and myself incorporated our deepening personal exploration and understanding of pre- and perinatal psychology into the work at our training Institute in Dartmoor England, the Karuna Institute. Along with this, I attended osteopathic college and was deeply touched by the cranial courses taught, where the heart of the work seemed to be about presence and perception, rather than analysis and doing.

In the early 1990s myself and two graduates from our Craniosacral training program, opened up a free baby clinic one day a week in Totnes, Devon, UK. We were seeing many single young mothers and their babies as well as some young families, incorporating both a pre- and perinatal psychology orientation and cranial approach to the healing work. One of my colleagues there was also an obstetrician, and his knowledge was often so helpful. What was obvious from the start of the clinic was that the work was so delicately poised, as we held both mother and baby in their processes with empathy and heart-centered exploration.

One thing that was also so clear was that the baby had his or her story to tell, and this needed to be heard, seen and received as their story unfolded. We learned to model our receptivity of baby as a sentient being for mothers and fathers; to include baby in all conversations, and to help mother and father slow down as their baby's story unfolded. It was such a learning process for us all!

I remember one young single mother bringing her one-month old baby to see us. Her baby would not sleep at night, cried a lot and seemed inconsolable. We quickly learned to slow our own process down because, even if a baby is expressing sympathetic nervous system anger and anxiety, their neurophysiology is much slower than adults, so that in part, our role was to help baby come into present time, feel safe again and to gradually co-regulate relationally with her mother.

In the first few sessions, we worked with both mother and baby, helping their systems regulate and come into a slower, more resourced relationship. We worked with baby's left-over birth process, which was certainly a story she needed to tell, and helped her resolve some of the remaining birthing forces in her system as well as helping her clear much of her emotional activation from that experience. After five or six sessions, her baby was much more settled, was sleeping much better and mother was relieved and much more resourced. We thought that much of the trauma that the baby had experienced during birth, which included being taken away from mum for a period of time in hospital, had cleared. However, a powerful thing happened some time later, which touched us all and was very humbling to observe.

Six months later, mother brought baby back for a 'check up'. Mother and baby knew us all and settled quickly, with baby smiling as she saw us. As the mother held her baby in her arms, one of the other therapists present contacted mother's thoracic area behind her heart, while I slowly made contact with baby's pelvic area. Baby first looked at me then turned and deeply looked at mom's eyes, made fists and, while crying angrily, started to strongly hit her mom. I knew how painful the birth process had been for them both. Mother had a relatively small pelvis and baby was full term and of a good size. It was a long and painful birth for mother, and her baby had been stuck for a period of time, experiencing strong pressures before forceps were used. She was then taken away for at least an hour before being brought back to mum. We now know how important it is after birth for a baby to come into contact with mother as soon as possible in order to securely bond and attach. I knew this history and said to baby, 'Yes it hurt you so much, but mum didn't mean to hurt you; it hurt her also.' Mum was crying and looked deeply into her daughter's eyes, holding her lovingly and said, 'Yes I didn't mean to hurt you, it hurt me too, so much!' She said this with such love, and then a wonderful thing occurred. Baby stopped crying in anger, stopped hitting mom, smiled and literally melted into her arms. It was a beautiful thing to be present for. I met mum and daughter almost a year later, and mum told me how wonderful their relationship had become. It was such a privilege to be present for this mutual healing process!

This book is a journey through this early territory not to be missed by clinicians of all kinds. We are beautifully introduced to the basics of early experience, its clinical, personal and interpersonal importance, with an overview of basic skills within the context of holding babies, mothers, families and adult clients in the exploration of the roots of their attachment processes, psychological health, personality development and safety-in-relationship. It also includes wonderful introductions to the neurophysiology of stress and health and how the nervous system develops and unfolds from the earliest times with relationship at its core. We are also introduced to the importance of knowing and sensing levels of activation that may arise in babies and adult process, with an introduction to appropriate trauma skills relative to the process arising. This is such important territory. The clinician must have the appropriate skills to help both babies and adult clients co-regulate, moderate and resolve their arising process in present-time. Along with all of this, there are clear descriptions of the clinical holding needed when working with babies and mothers, and the areas that may arise for holding, resolution and healing. Again I was so appreciative to see all of this included. Please, please slowly read and take all of it in! It is such a formative and important therapeutic and life journey!

Best wishes,
Franklyn Sills, MA, UKCP, RCST
Co-Director of the Karuna Institute, Devon, UK

ACKNOWLEDGEMENTS

I would like to thank all the contributors for giving their time and expertise so generously and the staff at Jessica Kingsley Publishers for allowing vital extra time to complete this book.

Translation: Felizitas Kafka, Andrea Braun, Stefanie Winkelbauer

Editing: Liz Hampson

Research: Jaana Tanilsoo

Images: George Baldwin

DISCLAIMER

The contents of this book are for information only and are not intended to replace or supersede professional medical advice. The authors and publishers admit no liability for any action or any claim howsoever arising from following any advice contained in this book. If you have any concerns about your health or medication, always consult your doctor. Readers must obtain their own professional medical advice before relying on or otherwise making use of any information contained in this book.

INTRODUCTION

John Wilks

This book is written for all therapists who work with babies and their families, whatever modality they use. It was not conceived as an instruction manual about specific techniques but is aimed more at providing a wide range of information about what we are dealing with when we work with babies and children, along with practical advice for working from a multidisciplinary and integrative perspective. All babies have been through an intense journey through conception, pregnancy and the process of birth and by the time they arrive at our clinic door they already have a myriad of different life stories to tell, and a host of different reasons why they might not be sleeping, feeding, digesting or progressing well.

Babies will bring not only the nuanced dynamics of family life but also their maternal and paternal generational history. They will bring the story of their pregnancy. How was it for them nutritionally, emotionally and even spiritually? Was the womb a safe place to be? How was the birth? It might have been easy for the mum, but was it easy for the baby? How were they welcomed into this world? All these elements might have been experienced in a positive or negative way, or a combination of the two, but rarely indifferently. They form the way babies perceive and relate to their environment and to us as therapists.

Experiences of pregnancy and birth form strengths and resources to be taken forward into adulthood; but they also have the potential to create 'dis-ease' and disease states both physically and psychologically. By addressing these at such a young age, we can go a long way to mitigate negative effects later in life. The issues we can help with are explored in this book and range from emotional, psychological and developmental to the physical. From clinical experience, impacts from pregnancy and birth affect every aspect of someone's life if not addressed. This can be as straightforward as a distortion in the temporomandibular joint (TMJ) as a result of birth trauma leading to a lifetime of dental work, to compression in the temporal area as a result of forceps causing a propensity for headaches, to subtler psychological imprinting of life statements such as 'I am not good enough', 'I always have to struggle' or 'there is never enough time'.

One of the major themes in this book is that it is much more important for us to create the right space in ourselves and in our clinic setting to work with babies rather than what we 'do' to a baby. Generally speaking, by the time babies come to us they will already have had a lot of things 'done to them' such as interventions at birth, premature removal from their mother, and a whole range of prenatal and postnatal tests. For us to be able to create a space where they can settle and tell their story is key without the need to rush to 'fix' them.

Babies are highly relational beings. They depend on relationship for their survival. So our abilities to settle ourselves, relate from our hearts, listen without judgement and empathize are all cornerstones of this work.

Common themes when working with babies

There are common themes that run through this book which are explored from different perspectives by different contributors, all of whom have spent many years developing their sophisticated approaches to working with babies and families. Many of the treatment approaches described here also apply to adults because adults carry their own 'baby history' with them. As we will see, one of the features of working with babies is how the birth histories of mothers and fathers get triggered and recapitulated when becoming parents themselves. It is essential to understand and recognize this when working with families as it affects the whole family dynamic and the baby's ability to feel safe and heard within that. Often a baby's distress is not so much related to its own physical discomfort but to a disturbance in the family 'field'. This is discussed in Chapter 5, 'Every Baby Has a Story to Tell', by Matthew Appleton.

For the therapist, some of the key features to bear in mind when working with babies and their families are:

- The need to create a sense of safety and containment in the therapy room when working with babies. From the viewpoint of attachment theory, safety is the primary thing babies need to feel in any situation, and is an essential prerequisite for doing any kind of therapeutic work. This is discussed in Chapters 7 and 8 by David Haas and Chapter 4 by Graham Kennedy.

- The need to include an awareness of the dynamics of the pregnancy for both mum and baby and to work towards acknowledging, hearing the story and healing that. There is a growing awareness in the pre- and perinatal field of the importance of prenatal factors (as opposed to focusing entirely on difficulties around birth) in later health outcomes. This is explored in Chapter 2 by Franz Ruppert and Chapter 1 by Ann Weinstein and Michael Shea.

- The need to work with empathy and from the heart. Research has shown that babies are highly attuned to resonate with their mother's heart field (Shea 2007). Ways of encouraging more coherence between mother and baby are discussed in Chapter 11 by Thomas Harms.

- Avoidance of the tendency to want to 'fix' things or even 'make them better' for parents or babies. If we try and fix things for a baby, then our agenda can over-ride that of the baby. Her priorities might not be the same as ours or even her parents.

- The need to give plenty of time for babies to tell their story. Babies need time to settle into a therapeutic relationship, some more than others. To rush them would be like an adult meeting someone for the first time and expecting them to tell you their most intimate problems. It doesn't help if there is pressure from the person listening.

- The importance of managing maternal stress levels when treating mums. Stress, particularly the consequences of long-term stress, is discussed in Chapter 1 by Ann Weinstein and Michael Shea.

- Understanding the importance of prenatal influences when treating symptoms such as colic, poor feeding or sleeping problems. Colic may be down to a number of factors such as the development of the microbiome (discussed in Chapter 9 by Carolyn Goh) and/or umbilical issues (discussed in Chapter 6 by Matthew Appleton).

Even when treating teenagers or adults, symptoms such as abdominal migraines can be related to maternal stress during pregnancy.

- Understanding the interrelationship of developing gut health and the development of the autonomic nervous system, particularly the vagus nerve.

- The importance of understanding Polyvagal Theory and the social engagement system, especially when treating premature babies in relation to factors such as eye contact and exposure to noise in the therapy room. This is referred to in various chapters, specifically Chapter 3 by Carolyn Goh.

- How generational factors affect babies, particularly how trauma can be passed on through both paternal and maternal lines, as discussed in Chapters 7 and 8 by David Haas.

- The effects of interventions at birth such as induction, Caesarean section, pain-relieving drugs and forceps. This is explored in my chapter (Chapter 10) and is multi-factorial. All interventions will have physical effects (compression, intra-osseous patterns, inflammation, etc.) but will also have psychological ramifications. Even powerful belief systems and life-statements such as 'life is painful' or 'things are done to me without me being asked – I don't have any say in decision-making' can arise at this time.

- The effects of various types of medication such as antibiotics and antidepressants on both the baby in the womb and postnatally in terms of symptoms such as allergies, digestive problems, immune system health and restlessness.

- The importance of very careful negotiation around therapeutic touch, particularly in areas where babies have met with difficulty in the birth process.

- The importance of a therapist not jumping to conclusions too quickly about what is happening in a therapy session with babies. Very often, what a baby is bringing to the session is not just 'one thing' such as the residual effects of forceps, but is often a series of related events that compound one another. For example, a baby who was subject to an attempted termination may have strong issues with trust and self-worth so that a later painful intervention can reinforce feelings of being 'bad' or being 'not good enough'.

Some factors, such as tongue-tie, primitive reflexes and breastfeeding, are touched on only briefly in this book, partly because they are all huge subjects in their own right, but also because they have already been written about extensively elsewhere. Likewise, the many environmental, nutritional and pharmacological influences on pregnancy and the newborn are not discussed in detail as they were covered in my previous book Choices in Pregnancy and Childbirth. More recent, and sometimes worrying associations between developmental issues and the use of SSRIs in pregnancy, the microbiome's influence on the development of the vagus nerve, and the potential link between paracetamol use (for example when used in conjunction with vaccinations) and autism are touched on in Chapter 9 but would benefit from further research by the reader.

There is an assumption in this book that babies are highly tuned social beings, conscious of their surroundings and the emotional state of their caregivers, that they are highly sensitive to touch and remember every aspect of the pregnancy and birth. From my own personal experience, which is validated by the work of such pioneers as David Chamberlain (2013) and Thomas Verny (2014), I would take this further and state that babies clearly remember landmarks like conception, implantation and even the pre-conception journey. My introduction to this work started with complete scepticism about the impact of these events on later health outcomes, but I had to eat my words as I became more and more aware of extremely early patterns emerging in the therapy room, both in observations of babies' body language and behaviour and my own powerful revelations during regression work.

The wounded therapist

One of the aspects that has become very clear for those working in the field of pre- and perinatal psychology, and particularly for those working actively with babies and parents, is the need for us, as therapists, to try and heal our own early history. Many of us are drawn into this work because of our early trauma history and we can have a strong desire to 'make it better' for people (babies included). Although this can be a powerful incentive for doing good in the world, it can, in a strange way, make our work less effective as we try to 'rescue' the people we are working with. This need to rescue often comes from a place of deep wounding in ourselves, and that place has its own history and its own agenda which can be at odds with those we are trying to help.

From a psychotherapeutic perspective, many of us became rescuers because we needed to ensure that our primary caregiver survived. We may have prioritized their survival to the detriment of our own well-being. As you will see from Chapter 1 by Ann Weinstein and Michael Shea, this tendency can even start in the womb and is hardwired in us in order to ensure our own survival. Issues related to survival patterns can be very hard to break or to even recognize in us, as they begin at such an early stage in our development. They are almost instilled in our tissues and become part of 'who we are'. To give up being a rescuer can in some way feel quite dangerous and threatening to us because at some time in our lives we may have had to put our own needs second in order to survive. This is why it is so important for therapists to look at their own patterns of behaviour. Beginning to look at these tendencies can be a challenging but an extraordinarily rich journey. The more we realize how these ingrained patterns of behaviour rule every aspect of our lives, the better therapists we become. Even if we can't change these patterns, we can at least bring them into awareness. It's a strange conundrum that the more we want to make it better for our clients the more we can 'get in the way' of deep healing.

Working on our tolerance levels for being able to hold distress is also very important. It can be very challenging working with babies and parents who are inconsolable, and the need to try and fix this *now* can engender feelings of helplessness and powerlessness in a therapist, in the same way that it can create feelings of inadequacy in parents. It can set therapists up for failure and shame. Life statements such as 'I am a bad therapist' are familiar territory for people working in the pre- and perinatal field. David Haas explains why they are such strong triggers for us as therapists as they can key into these very early pre-verbal memories of shame, 'badness' and failure. Thomas Harms describes an approach to working with babies who are inconsolable that he has developed over many years in Germany; it stresses the need for increasing tolerance levels in both parents and therapists.

The fact is that it is very difficult to hold a safe space for babies if we are constantly triggered into our own trauma patterns from our own birth or early history. Supervision and therapy are essential to do our work properly. This work is challenging but hugely enriching at the same time. It is very clear from all the research in this area that it is essential for all health professionals to grasp a deep understanding of the ramifications of how babies come into this world and to bring much more sensitivity and awareness into the way we treat babies and their mothers. This is vital if we are going to heal future generations, as the factors around pregnancy and birth impact physiologically, emotionally and psychologically incrementally on future generations. The future emotional and physical health of our grandchildren and our great-grandchildren is in our hands now.

Outline of the book

Because of the nature of an edited book with different contributors, there is a small amount of overlap in subject matter, but portrayed from different perspectives. Deciding on an order of chapters was not easy, and readers may feel inclined to change the order in which they read this book.

Some of the core principles and background information about prenatal stress, the social nervous system, bonding and attachment theory are presented towards the beginning of the book as they provide the theoretical foundation for what comes later in terms of practical treatment approaches.

We begin by looking at prenatal influences on health outcomes with chapters by Ann Weinstein and Michael Shea, and Franz Ruppert. Carolyn Goh then looks at the science behind what is called the 'social engagement system' particularly regarding the vagus nerve and its role in regulating physiological responses in babies. We then go on to explore bonding and attachment behaviour as outlined by Graham Kennedy before looking at types of crying and babies' body language with Matthew Appleton.

David Haas describes a model of working with families and babies that outlines practical strategies for working within babies' and parents' tolerance levels. We then move on with Carolyn Goh to the gut from the perspective of the baby's developing immune system and microbiome as well as looking at prenatal umbilical issues in relation to symptoms such as 'colic'. There follows a chapter looking at the ramifications for treatment for babies who have experienced pharmacological and mechanical interventions at birth. Thomas Harms describes methods of working with inconsolable babies in a crisis situation which he calls 'Emotional First Aid', and the book finishes with an overview of some of the different treatment approaches currently used with babies.

At the end of the book is a resources section giving further information and details of available training courses. For any therapist whose interest is whetted by the information in this book, I would strongly recommend taking classes from the perspectives of both personal development and practical applications for working with babies. There are now a number of courses out there that therapists, midwives, doulas, doctors and health visitors can attend to deepen their understanding of this work. These are listed at the end of this book.

Terminology

Because this book contains contributors from the UK, Germany and the USA it adopts both UK and North American spelling and terminology. Babies are variously referred to as infants, he or she depending on the contributor's preference.

References

Chamberlain, D.B. (2013) *Windows to the Womb: Revealing the Conscious Baby from Conception to Birth.* Berkeley, CA: North Atlantic Books.

Shea, M.J. (2007) *Biodynamic Craniosacral Therapy* (Vol. 1). Berkeley, CA: North Atlantic Books.

Verny, T.R. (2014) 'What cells remember: Toward a unified field theory of memory.' *Journal of Prenatal & Perinatal Psychology & Health 29*, 1, 16–28.

CHAPTER 1

STRESS DURING PREGNANCY

FETAL-PLACENTAL MECHANISMS AND ANTIDOTES

Ann Diamond Weinstein, PhD, and Michael J. Shea, PhD

Introduction

Biology is narrative. This chapter discusses pregnancy and fetal-placental development in light of new research on maternal stress. We are calling for a new understanding of how pregnant mothers and their families are treated during this sacred time of life. During pregnancy, a bridge is formed between a woman's or girl's biology and her emerging narrative or story of her pregnancy. It now appears that the placenta takes on functions that were typically thought to be unique to the central nervous system, such as the capability of receiving, processing, and acting upon a wide variety of external stimuli. Thus the placenta plays a very important role and is designed to act on behalf of the fetus as both a sensory and motor organ. It acts as a transducer and integrator of environmental signals into the developmental process of the fetus epigenetically. This will be explained below. The developmental process of the baby can thus be profoundly impacted in terms of long-term health and well-being from maternal stress. Thus attention must and should be placed on the mom since her biology can manifest as sensation, feelings, emotions, and different states of mind.

Recent research has identified prenatal stress as a very serious detriment to the immediate and long-term health and well-being of the embryo, fetus, infant, and adult (Danese and McEwen 2012; Lupien *et al.* 2009; Sandman and Davis 2012; Shonkoff, Boyce, and McEwen 2009; Van den Bergh *et al.* 2005; Wadhwa 2005; Wadhwa *et al.* 2002, 2011). Many women and girls report experiencing high levels of stress in their lives and feel they have little time and limited resources they can use to fulfill their needs in healthy ways. Researchers Wadhwa *et al.* (2011) explain that stress is a 'person–environment interaction, in which there is a perceived discrepancy between environmental demands and the individual's psychological, social or biological resources'. Direct links have been made between prenatal maternal mood and fetal behavior, as well as significant genetic adaptations in the human placenta from different types of stress (Monk, Spicer, and Champagne 2012; Myatt 2006; Wadhwa *et al.* 2001).

Some pregnant women and girls have experienced past or recent severe stress and trauma. Robert Scaer, an expert in the field of trauma, notes that during a traumatic experience, severe stress escalates to the point where an individual feels her life is threatened. A feeling of helplessness is also a key component of traumatic experience (Scaer 2007, 2012). These pregnant women and girls may experience traumatic stress symptoms and post-traumatic stress disorder (PTSD) during pregnancy which may be associated with pregnancy complications that impact the health and development of their offspring (Yehuda *et al.* 2005), including their birthweight and length of gestation (Seng *et al.* 2011). PTSD will be discussed below.

Some mothers experience a state of chronic stress. This can include the stress induced by a diet that provides inadequate maternal nutrition, which modifies the physiology and metabolism of the pregnant and postpartum mother, and programs the fetus for heart disease later in life (Saad *et al.* 2016). Cigarette smoking and exposure to second-hand smoke are also very stressful on the embryo and fetus and are linked to childhood obesity (Durand, Logan, and Carruth 2007), anxiety and cardiovascular disease (see CDC 2016 for a complete list of the effects of smoking during pregnancy).

Stress may also be triggered intermittently by any event in the external or internal environment of the mother. Stephen Porges (2004) coined the term 'neuroception' to describe how an individual, in microseconds and beneath conscious awareness, perceives and reacts to their internal and/or external environment. The specific psychophysiological states associated with the neuroception of environmental safety, danger, or life threat are expressed in an individual's neuroendocrine, cardiovascular, and immune systems. If a mother's neuroception of her environment evokes an experience of safety, her social engagement system will be activated. When a mother's neuroception of her internal and/or external environment evokes an experience of danger, fight-or-flight responses will be activated. When her neuroception of her internal and/or external environment evokes an experience of life threat, freeze/dissociation/shutdown behaviors will be activated. It must be pointed out that in a clinical setting, the establishment of safety is of critical importance when working with a pregnant mom.

Epigenetics and morphology

Embryonic-fetal growth and development are influenced by two dynamics. The first is the expression of one's epigenetic influences (Holt and Patterson 2006). There is a sleeve around the DNA in the cell nucleus that signals when to switch on and switch off optimal genes during development. The sleeve around the DNA is divided into zones depending on what is being built by the cell. It is like a sheet of music specifying which note is played and when it is played. The switching can be influenced by a mother's psycho-emotional state or even by the last meal she ate. If there is a stress influence, a less optimal gene may be expressed from the particular zone being targeted. This is the science of epigenetics in brief.

The second influential dynamic of growth and development is from the morphology (the physical and fluid movement) of cells, cell aggregates, individual structures within embryos, the whole form of the embryo and the fetus. All cells in the body are interconnected via fluid communication systems with a substrate of, firstly, biological water and, secondly, the blood. In addition, there are signaling proteins in each cell that connect with every cell in the body like an interstate highway system. Therefore, epigenetics and morphology are partners in the dance of development throughout our lifespan, but especially prenatally. Both involve movement at a microscopic and whole-body level. At the level of the whole body, a woman may begin to sense the enormity of her and her baby's metabolism.

The epigenetic process may be an evolutionary attempt, as imperfect as it is, by the developing organism to prepare for, or adapt to the environment based on environmental exposures of the past and present. In a way, there are no perfectly optimal growth vectors because the human organism is constantly adapting, which is natural. However, bringing forward transgenerational family imprinting can be a less than optimal adaptation. At the same time the embryo and fetus is responding to the natural world in the present moment. Although the human embryo has similarities in its development, every human embryo has different time lines for the differentiation of structures and functions. This means that the term *optimal* has a wide range of possibilities, as does the term *normal* or *natural*.

Stress imprinting

The mother's body–mind equilibrium is essential during pregnancy and she needs support to become more conscious of such equilibrium. It is vital that the care provided to the mother assists her in developing stress reduction skills that may reduce the negative impacts of stress on her embryo and fetus-placenta, including the influence of stress on the expression of genes (epigenetics) in the embryo and fetus-placenta. This type of support or education must be based on loving kindness rather than fear. The negative impacts of stress and traumatic stress include pregnancy complications such as intrauterine growth restriction (IUGR) and premature birth (Wadhwa *et al.* 2001, 2011). IUGR (which is discussed below) is associated with epigenetic switching, which also causes a wide variety of other challenges during pregnancy, birth, and the postpartum period (Hunt 2006; Huppertz *et al.* 2006; Sibley *et al.* 2005).

Stress imprinting (epigenetic imprinting) can occur at any time in the lifespan of an egg or a sperm, from the time when the egg first differentiated (when the mother herself was an embryo in her mother's womb), during the mom and dad's adolescence, and all the way up through ovulation and fertilization. Every egg is different in this way, as are sperm. Some eggs could be 'hibernating' in the ovaries for 30 years with an imprint, and others might not get imprinted until ovulation. No two eggs are the same, and the same imprint does not occur in the egg immediately adjacent to it. And, yes, it is the same process with the sperm cell. So again, what is optimal for one embryo and fetus may be quite different for another, even in identical twins.

Fetal programming

Because numerous diseases have now been identified as having their origins in the fetal environment – diabetes, heart disease, hypertension, obesity, and others – a new scientific model of pregnancy has been developed. It is called the *fetal programming hypothesis* or stress vulnerability model (Wadhwa 2005). This model postulates that maternal stress during pregnancy impacts the in-utero environment and can alter the development of the fetus during particularly sensitive periods. This may also include a permanent effect on what is called the phenotype or the end expression of genetic inheritance. This typically shows up in low-birthweight babies or babies who are obese at birth or quickly become obese after birth (Gillman 2008; Whitaker 2004). The occurrence of low-birthweight babies has tripled in the past ten years according to the Harvard T.H. Chan School of Public Health (2016). What has not been revealed are effective measures to stem the tide of this epidemic. Haig (1993, 1996), an evolutionary biologist, refers to this as the 'struggle of pregnancy'. One common measurement is the cost to the health care system, which can be enormous in some disease processes. As much as stress imprinting and fetal programming may create a metabolic struggle in the mother, there is equally a system of cooperation, which will be discussed shortly.

Obesity has become particularly problematic in our culture. At its most basic, the term 'obesity' describes having too much body fat. The most commonly used measure of weight status is the body mass index, or BMI. BMI uses a simple calculation based on the ratio of one's height and weight. Determining one's BMI and its interpretation can readily be done on the internet. More recent research has shown that waist circumference and measurement of visceral fat to determine obesity also correlates well with important health outcomes such as heart disease, diabetes, cancer, and overall mortality. Pregnant moms can be obese along with their unborn babies. Low-birthweight babies can become obese shortly after birth as mentioned, indicating a significant metabolic problem established during or possibly before the pregnancy. Obese babies are now a growing concern because of dysregulated metabolism in the baby leading to the likelihood of metabolic syndromes such as diabetes, heart disease, and continued obesity through the lifespan. More children than ever before are manifesting heart disease.

Cited studies in this chapter on work-related stress and adverse pregnancy outcomes also show that occupational exposure is particularly associated with low birthweight, including physically demanding work, prolonged standing, shift and night work, and high levels of cumulative work fatigue. Physically demanding work is also related to pregnancy-induced hypertension and pre-eclampsia. Severe life events, such as the death of a family member, accidents, and illnesses, have been shown to increase the frequency of cranial neural crest malformations in the child (de la Cruz and Markwald 1998). This means that there will be a potential problem with the development of the heart and vascular system. It is now known that over half of all birth defects are in the heart and vascular system (Kirby 2007). Neural crest cells (the earliest cells in the embryo that differentiate to become the autonomic nervous system) play an important role in the development of the aorta and certain parts of the heart during the embryonic and fetal time of life (Tomanek and Runyan 2001). These authors point out that over half of all birth defects are defects of the cardiovascular system.

As a pregnancy progresses, rest–activity cycles related to the mother's own imprinting in her autonomic nervous system begin to be linked to specific fetal heart rate patterns, as well as to the absence or presence of rapid eye movements (REM) in the mother. Rapid eye movements are now known to be critical to getting a good night's sleep; with the epidemic of insomnia in contemporary society, one can easily trace some of these poor sleeping patterns to the prenatal time of life. Sleep is restorative to the whole body and nervous systems.

Fetal movement – ADHD

Along with heart rate patterns and eye movements, fetal movement patterns are important indicators of fetal states and development. There are between 11 and 16 basic fetal body movements. When a fetus does not make these movements there is a direct link to learning disabilities in childhood and adolescence as well as attention deficit disorders (Birnholz, Stephens, and Faria 1976). Research by Van den Bergh and Marcoen (2004) links maternal stress and ADHD (Attention Deficit Hyperactive Disorder) in eight- and nine-year-olds. The sleep and stress control systems share particular brain locations, such as the locus coeruleus and the prefrontal cortex. It is very difficult to think clearly and to self-regulate emotionally when under stress and unable to sleep.

Maternal PTSD

Pregnant moms with a history of traumatic stress symptoms or diagnosed PTSD are also particularly vulnerable to dysregulated autonomic states during pregnancy that may affect the growing fetus. Cited research in this chapter suggests that maternal anxiety and stress-related mechanisms affect the fetal nervous system during the first two trimesters of pregnancy.

Van den Bergh *et al.* (2005) conclude that the link between maternal prenatal emotional stress and later infant or child behavior persists even after controlling for different research biases and other dynamics that occur in the prenatal and postnatal period of life. Because of this, there is now a great deal of support for the fetal programming hypothesis due to maternal stress.

Cited research in this chapter further indicates that maternal anxiety during pregnancy is also significantly associated with challenges in infant orientation and autonomic nervous system stability. Greater activation of the right hemisphere has been demonstrated in the infant as well as elevated levels of cortisol and norepinephrine. Elevated levels of these neurotransmitters can be quite toxic to the fetal and infant brain (Sandman and Davis 2012). Along with these elevated levels, lower levels of dopamine and serotonin in the newborn have been found (Nathanielsz 1996). Women and girls may experience both PTSD and depression in the preconception, prenatal and early postnatal period. Infants of mothers with symptoms of depression tend to cry excessively after birth and are difficult to console. It is clear that children of depressed mothers show increased autonomic arousal, including higher heart rates and reduced activity in brain regions that mediate positive social relational behavior. The link between prenatal stress and regulation problems at the cognitive, behavioral, and emotional levels in the child has now been clearly identified.

Maternal freeze/dissociation, freeze/shutdown responses, and endogenous opioids

Women and girls with past experiences of trauma and/or traumatic stress symptoms may experience a felt sense of life threat in the preconception, prenatal, and early parenting periods. If they are pregnant, they may experience a felt sense of life threat for their developing baby as well. They may experience a lack of control and helplessness as their bodies change over the course of the pregnancy. This may also occur if they experience medical conditions and complications during the pregnancy, as well as during medical exams and procedures and interactions with health care practitioners. A neuroception (Porges 2004) of life threat may be triggered in pregnant women and girls long after a traumatic event(s) is over. This may also happen in women receiving reproductive endocrinology treatment for infertility.

The freeze/dissociation or freeze/shutdown response, which is triggered during a felt sense of life threat, manifests in behavioral and neuroendocrine stress system responses dominated by the parasympathetic branch of the autonomic nervous system. These differ from those evoked during a neuroception of danger, which triggers a fight-or-flight response that manifests in behavioral and neuroendocrine stress system responses dominated by the sympathetic branch of the autonomic nervous system. The freeze/dissociation, freeze/shutdown response is characterized by the release of endogenous opioids, including endorphins, enkephalins, and dynorphins (Lanius 2014). The fight-or-flight response is characterized by the release of epinephrine, norepinephrine, and corticotropin-releasing hormone (CRH) (Buckley 2015). As noted in the introduction to this chapter, a wealth of research demonstrates the impacts of these stress hormones on the fetus, infant, child, and adult. Minimal research has explored the impact of recurrent maternal freeze/dissociation, freeze/shutdown states and endogenous opioids on the developing embryo and fetus, and the maternal–placental–fetal relationship.

The reactivity of a mother's opioid system in response to stress and/or trauma and the frequency of her experiences of freeze/shutdown states shape the physiological environment in which her prenate grows. This, in turn, influences the development and programming of her offspring's stress response system and their response to stress and/or trauma over their lifespan. The impacts of prenatal exposure to high levels of maternal endogenous opioids may be associated with their synchronicity with critical periods of fetal brain development and the programming of the prenate's key regulatory systems (Thomson 2007; Wadhwa *et al.* 2011).

If a mother has experienced past or recent trauma and/or loss, including prenatal trauma during her gestation in her own mother's womb, and/or early childhood attachment trauma in interactions with her primary caregivers, her stress response system, including her opioid system, may have been shaped by these experiences and in turn may affect her interactions with her infant in the postnatal period, further influencing her infant's developing stress response system (Weinstein 2016). The effects of endogenous opioids include a reduction in the availability of sensory input, interference with the experience of emotion and the transmission of sensory information to the cortex, and the regulation of sensory input (Lanius 2014).

Endogenous opioids may also affect areas of the mother's brain that are involved with integrating body schema and depersonalization

(Simeon *et al.* 2009). The release of endogenous opioids during states of freeze/dissociation, freeze/shutdown serves to physically and emotionally disconnect the mother from distressing feelings associated with past trauma and/or loss that may be triggered by body changes during pregnancy and/or sensations related to the movement and growth of her prenate. This disconnection may inhibit the trauma survivor's capacity for interoception and her ability to connect with her baby before and after birth (Weinstein 2016).

The fetal–placental relationship

This leads to a discussion of the fetal–placental relationship. Because of prenatal maternal stress, the fetus undergoes what is called oxidative stress in the placenta. Oxidative stress is a reaction of the oxygen molecule to other toxic levels of molecules such as cortisol mentioned earlier. It splits off smaller oxygen molecules that interfere with metabolism. These smaller oxygen molecules are known as *free radicals* that are toxic to the intracellular environment. Consequently, cells have a very difficult time detoxifying their internal environment. This in turn damages the cell and its DNA. The most common example in the mineral world is rust (iron oxide) which no car or home owner wants. It is also seen as the brown on an apple that has been cut open. So, due to maternal stress, the placenta gets 'rusty' and cannot process the toxic rust, so to speak. The channels that normally carry waste products out into circulation and elimination are compromised.

The placenta itself is essentially a fetal endocrine gland and operates as the immune system of the fetus as well as part of its nervous system. The placenta also has its own cardiovascular system. Technically, the mother's cells in her blood do not go through the placenta but rather molecules of nutrition are extracted by the placental villi and placed into fetal circulation in the umbilical cord. However, some cells from the fetus do enter the mother's circulatory system and mom's cells can be found in her children as well. This will be discussed below.

What the fetus requires is nutritional fertilizer in the form of nutritive molecules coming directly from the umbilical vein for its heart. What the heart doesn't use is taken immediately by the brain and, finally, the remaining organs and tissues of the embryo and fetus. Thus there is a hierarchy of recipients of the mother's nutrition – the heart, the brain, and then everything else. All organ systems of the body have different developmental rates prenatally. This means that each organ system has critical periods unrelated to other organs so that the specific nutrition needs of the prenate, while varying constantly, must nevertheless have access to a rich regular supply from which to draw. The mother provides various molecules from her blood to help build the different systems of the body, including the immune system (Hunt 2006).

The placenta

The placenta is made up of four different kinds of villi. The *stem* villi provide a type of scaffolding or support framework. The *terminal* villi represent the principal sites of maternal–fetal exchange. There are also intermediate, *mature* villi and intermediate, *immature* villi. The intermediate villi are secondary sites of the maternal–fetal exchange. When there is elevated cortisol in the mother's blood, it creates stress in all of the villi and causes oxygen deprivation (hypoxia) related to pre-eclampsia (Karanam, Page, and Anim-Nyame 2010). Thus the maternal blood oxygen in the intervillous space of the placenta is dysregulated, causing oxidative stress, an inflammatory condition. This leads to depleted blood-nutrition factors entering the embryo-fetus and causing oxidative stress. Epigenetic changes begin to occur in the fetal-placental villi structure, which can be damaging to the fetus, resulting in an intensive medicalized birth, neonatal challenges, childhood developmental delays, or cardiovascular disease at any time in the lifespan. This is just the tip of the iceberg in terms of poor health outcomes (Relier 2001).

In general, during the second week post-fertilization, the trophoblast (outer mantle of cells surrounding the embryo or pre-placenta) and its ultimate structure weeks later, the placenta, express the genes of the father, while the embryo expresses the genes of the mother, especially in the nervous system. These specific parental genes are imprinted genes, which means that if a paternally derived gene that is supposed to be switched on in the placenta is repressed because of placental insufficiency and reduced fetal growth, an altered expression of the placental gene will occur, because the silent maternal gene will turn on instead. Likewise, the maternal genes of the embryo must be turned on normally, and if the silent paternal gene is switched on epigenetically in the embryo, less than optimal outcomes are likely to follow. It is now thought that such dysregulation of the maternal and paternal genes ultimately result in disease processes. The placenta begins to change its phenotype and structure (Myatt 2006), as does the embryo-fetus due to inflammatory conditions.

An inflammatory placenta from oxidative stress and an altered uterine blood flow filled with too many stress hormones and stress neurotransmitters will lead to different fetal-placental expressions of their unique structure and function discussed shortly. Not only will there be the long-term health problems as partially outlined above, but also a significant aberration in healthy, normal birth weight. Low-birthweight babies can be tremendously challenging, as evident in neonatal intensive care units (Sibley *et al.* 2005).

Intrauterine growth restriction (IUGR)

Because the placenta actively regulates the nature and extent of nutrient transfer to the fetus, any inflammation due to stress can compromise the fetus to a greater or lesser extent with delayed health consequences that might show up right after birth, or not until decades later. This process results in IUGR (Brodsky and Christou 2004). IUGR is the failure of a fetus to reach its growth potential and is thus associated with a poor health outcome, particularly in the neonatal period, and especially in premature infants. The impairment of fetal-placental circulation in the villi and the consequent decrease in the ability of the fetus to extract oxygen are of great importance because the centers of the brain that monitor oxygen are developing in the limbic system. Hypoxia is a determining factor in the growth of the brain and the vasculature feeding the brain during pregnancy and neonatally (Andreone, Lacoste, and Gu 2015). Hypoxia could be a risk factor for anxiety and panic disorders later in life, so it makes sense for therapists to help coach a pregnant mom with her breathing.

Of great interest in infant research is the effect on the development of the brain, especially the prefrontal cortex, of different styles of attachment between a mother and her baby. The prefrontal cortex and its many subdivisions have extensive and reciprocal connections with all the sensory systems, especially the arousal and attention functions throughout the limbic, midbrain, and brain stem areas. Functions such as motivation, drive, and appropriate self-regulation responses from stimuli are key to the importance of the prefrontal cortex. IUGR, however, causes greater blood flow to the brain stem of the developing fetus and thus potentially reinforces survival-oriented responses to life situations. The brain stem is considered to be the more primitive part of the brain. If the prefrontal cortex is deprived of nutrient-rich blood in the fetus, the potential for resilience and self-regulation is reduced and the potential for aggression and violence during the lifespan is increased.

Corticotropin-releasing hormone (CRH)

Much research has been done on the development of the fetal nervous system and brain. Elevated cortisol is now linked to elevated placental CRH (Wadhwa 2005). At this level of fetal challenge, the maternal–placental–fetal neuroendocrine axis is disrupted. The main culprit in poor neonatal outcomes seems to be placental CRH. Placental CRH is identical to adult hypothalamic CRH. It plays a crucial role in regulating human reproductive biology and modulation of maternal and fetal pituitary-adrenal function. This also includes participation in fetal cellular differentiation, growth, and maturation, and *the physiology of birth*. Common to maternal stress is elevated maternal and placental CRH. This is a set-up for low thresholds of resilience later in life as well as stress-related disorders due to dysregulated autonomic nervous systems.

When the placenta generates too much CRH, the fetus-placenta begins a biological struggle with the mother to get its needs met. It will secrete hormones to increase mom's blood pressure to get more nutrition. The mom's endocrine system will actively attempt to suppress the flow to the placenta. This is the metabolic struggle mentioned earlier. But it is also, at the same time, adapting and attempting to cooperate, particularly through the process of 'microchimerism', which is a term discussed later. All these factors are present. But above all, the embryo and fetus, the infant and child, as well as the mother, are highly vulnerable to metabolic and physiological insult, especially at these fundamental levels of the endocrine and immune system regulatory hormones. Stress reduction strategies for every pregnant mom must be available via early intervention programs which, ideally, offer a variety of options such as prenatal yoga, pregnancy massage, acupuncture, or other forms of relaxing, somatic-based therapy. Sometimes just having child care for a period of time can allow the parents to destress. Germany has a program as part of its socialized medicine in which parents can spend a weekend at a spa with full child care at no expense to the parents.

Throughout life, the experiences that we have with other people, our family of origin, and the natural world help form the heart, brain, and body. A body narrative is formed by the internal and external environment. It has long been known that cortisol in elevated levels is dangerous to the brain and is related to long-term negative effects in behavior and cognitive development. Fetal exposure to cortisol and its stimulation of placental CRH directly affects the development and function of critical neurotransmitter systems in the brain stem and decreases the connections of the prefrontal cortex to the amygdala via the insular cortex.

The amygdala, the fear center of the brain, may become more dominant without the mediating effects of the self-regulatory functions of the prefrontal cortex. Likewise, the heart is directly linked to the amygdala for survival during trauma, and even this relationship is dysregulated; the heart overreacts to non-noxious stimuli, creating a cascade of neurological overwhelming events resulting in a perceived lack of safety. When such a lack of safety is imprinted on the fetus prenatally, its development after birth can be greatly compromised. Likewise, the mother can have difficulty responding appropriately to non-threatening stimuli as she may perceive such stimuli as fearful and threatening.

Hypothalamic–pituitary–adrenal–thyroid–gonadal (HPATG) axis

Fetal programming of the important HPATG axis and other important functional relationships between the brain, the heart, and the endocrine system can occur. The HPATG axis is controlled by the prefrontal cortex and is a likely candidate for many of the regulation problems seen at the cognitive, behavioral, and emotional level in children whose mothers suffered with anxiety and stress during pregnancy. Thus, it is more than likely that fetal programming of the HPATG axis, limbic system, and prefrontal cortex contributes to the epidemic of regulation problems found in children of mothers who are highly stressed during pregnancy, have a history of post-traumatic stress disorder (PTSD), or experience current traumatic stress symptoms and/or depression.

One of the primary alterations is the *set point* of the HPATG axis. Such metabolic adaptations that enable the fetus to adapt to prenatal stress and loss of nutrition result in the permanent reprogramming of the developmental pattern within key tissue and organ systems in the fetus. This has clear pathological consequences in the adult, primarily in the domain of metabolic syndromes such as heart disease, obesity, and diabetes, but also numerous behavioral and cognitive challenges. This model of *fetal programming* suggests that humans are much more vulnerable to an unhealthy and adverse uterine environment than other species. One reason for this is because human cell division occurs much more rapidly in the womb than in other animal species. How much of these biological processes filter through to her conscious awareness?

A new paradigm

What is missing in our culture is a unifying new paradigm of pregnancy support. This is a moral challenge for our culture to provide more compassionate care for pregnant moms and their families. It is important to develop a new understanding of early development in which the embryo-fetus is seen as playing an active role in its own construction by evolving systems designed to acquire and use information throughout the lifespan regarding the nature of the environment (Hrdy 1999). He or she is a sentient human being. It is the environment that is guiding development in conjunction with innate factors of embryonic and fetal biology. The environment can be quite negative and/or there can be an organic problem with the embryo or fetus that is pre-existing. All this is happening within the woman's or girl's body. It is a lot to hold in our contemporary society without support.

Prematurity is the leading cause of infant mortality and significant health problems in the United States. The rate of prematurity is higher in the U.S. than in any other developed nation in the world and it has not decreased much in the past 40 years. Of the many problems with prematurity, low birth weight or what is called *birth phenotype* is the most critical. As discussed, fetal programming refers to the process by which conditions during crucial and sensitive periods of embryonic and fetal life have permanent effects on the structure and function of the human body, its physiology and metabolism. This early programming creates what are called *metabolic set points*, which define the behavioral, cognitive, and overall organismic dynamic of the adaptive range within which individuals can live, become more whole, and uncover within themselves an inherent completeness in which flaws are held in their wholeness. This adaptive range influences the susceptibility to disease process and is realized through numerous interactions with the world in which the infant, child, and adult live. Any and all persons who work with pregnant moms and their families must do so with mindfulness and compassion. Making a compassionate connection with pregnant moms, and all people for that matter, acknowledges a fundamental aspect of health that is unperturbed by fetal programming.

Innate compassion

As mentioned earlier, there is new literature on fetal-maternal cell trafficking called microchimerism. Fetal cells can cross through the placental barrier into the mother and vice versa. The emerging field of Fetal Maternal Microchimerism is an elegant example of biological compassion (Boddy *et al.* 2015; Kallenbach, Johnson, and Bianchi 2011; Mahmood and O'Donoghue 2014; Rijnink *et al.* 2015). In what researchers call a *metabolism of cooperation*, cells from the developing embryo and fetus enter the mother's bloodstream and gravitate towards her heart, brain, liver, and breasts. These cells are now known to have a healing effect on the mother when she experiences problems in those areas of her body. The fetal cells offer the mother protection from breast cancer and a reduced risk of rheumatoid arthritis. Fetal cells can also alert the immune system of the mother for the purpose of healing her heart. More than a system of cooperation, it is a *system of compassion* rooted in the cells of the mother's and child's bodies. It is an easy step to take, that this innate biological instinct for compassion could manifest behaviorally, psychologically, and spiritually through the lifespan. Compassion is our pre-existing cellular condition.

Conclusion and 'Compassion Connection'

Certain psychological challenges, as well as long-term problems that clients have with the central nervous system, the cardiovascular system, and the immune and endocrine systems, are now known to be directly linked to maternal stress during pregnancy. Research cited in this chapter has shown that the effects of prenatal stress may be more important than imprinting from a traumatic medicalized birth. This is because birth is the consequence of the entire prenatal time, a recapitulation of the preceding nine months and even earlier in terms of transgenerational imprinting. Research is indicating a more direct link between challenges during infancy and early childhood with fetal-placental development rather than birth processes. This is a very important point to consider in light of the current prenatal and perinatal psychological therapies focused on reliving and remembering *birth imprinting*. The pre- and perinatal field (PPN) needs to begin integrating and treating the underlying dynamic in the prenatal and/or preconception time of life that may have caused such a traumatic birth to occur or other adverse health outcomes. This means focusing on pregnant women and girls, lowering their stress and providing compassionate care for relieving fetal programming and embryonic imprinting.

An antidote is needed. It is vitally important that our culture learns to support mothers and families to optimize the health of the future of this planet. What is necessary is the development of mindfulness and compassion-based therapies that can access this prenatal and preconception dynamic in a more direct biological way, such as Biodynamic Cardiovascular Therapy and Mindfulness Based Childbirth and Parenting (MBCP). Our program for therapists to consider teaching to, and learning from, pregnant moms is called 'Compassion Connection'.

Compassion Connection

1. *Connect with Body.* The biology and physiology of pregnancy is complex, and if mothers are unable to get services such as massage, yoga, or acupuncture then they can *first* learn *Coherent Breathing 666*: six seconds of an inhale, six seconds of an exhale, for six minutes at a time, anywhere or anytime, sitting or lying down. Instructions for this type of breathing are readily available on the internet as well as the availability of numerous apps. Rasanen *et al.* (1998) demonstrated the vital importance of maternal breathing.

   Second, cardioception is interoceptive awareness of the movement of the heart. Simply sensing the movement of the heart gradually changes brain structure and brain chemistry by reducing fear and increasing resilience. Pregnant moms can learn to sense their own heart or take their pulse, which directly influences the fetal heart rate and improves the well-being of the baby.

Third, connecting with nature is important. Pregnant moms are well advised to spend time walking or sitting still in nature to improve health outcomes.

As discussed above in the section on maternal PTSD, pregnant women and girls with past experiences of trauma and/or loss may find it difficult to connect with their bodies as they may experience defense system responses and psychophysiological states of anxiety, fear, guilt, grief, and shame triggered by their changing bodies and the physical sensations associated with the growth and movement of their prenate. Sensitive care provided by a knowledgeable, skilled, compassionate practitioner is needed to support these mothers in experiencing a felt sense of safety while exploring connections with their bodies and their babies in the prenatal and postnatal periods (Weinstein 2016).

2. *Connect with Baby.* One antidote can be the telling of an *origin story*. However, a therapist might ask first: 'Are you comfortable talking to your child?' This starting point for the story is what is fresh right now for the mother. There needs to be respect for the first arising in the mom's experience in the moment. It is the first chapter in the origin story. As part of an intake, mom can also tell a story of how the pregnancy began, including its progression, to her unborn child. It is just like reading a bedtime story to the child. Either story comes from the heart and empowers the unborn child to differentiate its feelings from mom's feelings and for the mom to differentiate her feelings from her baby. The story can be told in segments over time. It can be told as an origin story by introducing the mother's whole family history or from conception forward or from right now as the starting point. Szejer (2005) insists that the baby be told the whole story as soon as possible.

Another story to tell might be the *mom's biography*, so the baby can get to know the mom. Another story could be *current events* in mom's life or the sensation in *mom's body* during pregnancy. The body story is a big story and can be helped tremendously with different forms of manual therapy. No matter what category of story being told, it is about mom letting her baby know that even with her stress, her baby is not responsible for such stress and mom will take care of it. 'I'm okay, you're okay' is the guiding principle and plot line in the story. It is essential that the therapist who facilitates the telling of the story has the capacity and skill to provide a quality of presence that supports a *safe* and *compassionate* container for both the mother's *and* the baby's experiences.

It is also essential that the therapist be able to observe and understand maternal signs of psychophysiological dysregulation during this process and support the mother in regulating her state to minimize potential negative impacts on her prenate. Education and training in therapeutic modalities that facilitate autonomic nervous system regulation are vital when working with pregnant moms and their babies.

Pregnant women and girls may experience a wide range of feelings about their developing babies, which are shaped by their lived experiences from their own conception to the present. We now understand that there is also the potential for the transgenerational transmission of trauma from one generation to another. Therefore, experiences of previous generations may also shape a mother's feelings and experiences during her pregnancy with her own child. The preconception period is the optimal time to address transgenerational imprints and anticipatory feelings related to pregnancy.

If the woman or girl is currently pregnant, the therapist is there to help the mom to differentiate between her past experiences that have shaped her current experience of this pregnancy and this prenate, and to access a felt sense of this developing baby's unique, individual nature and essence. This is a discovery process for the story teller and the story listener. It is a ritual of inclusion in which an unborn baby can be recognized as having a sense of belonging or simply being here. A mom is encouraged to share from the heart.

Some mothers may hold adverse or conflicted feelings about the experience of being pregnant and the presence of their prenate within. These feelings may include fear, shame, anger, and repulsion among others, depending on her experiences prior to the pregnancy. If these feelings arise, then they are to be respected as part of the mother's experience. It is crucial that these feelings be differentiated from the unborn, so he or she does not internalize the mother's adverse feelings as qualities of being that inherently belong to them. The context in which this occurs along with the quality of the mother's communication and the vulnerability of the prenate as receiver of these communications must be considered.

In addition, it is important that the therapist follows up with the mother in the days and weeks after this experience to provide the mother with an opportunity to express any feelings she might have as she reflects on the story-telling process. This may also provide an opportunity for her to connect with a felt sense of her prenate's feelings following the story-telling experience. This is particularly important if the mother expressed adverse or conflicted feelings about her experience of pregnancy and the presence of her prenate. Whatever story arises, the mom is always telling the story to her baby first and then to others who are there to listen.

Another way to connect with the unborn child is to feel its heart and vascular system. Mom can use her hands to explore the location of the fetal heart rate via different locations of the cardiac pulse. Mom may simply be able to sense the cardiovascular system of her baby. Blood volume increases 50 percent in a woman's body while pregnant. Can mom feel the heartbeat of her child? Can mom palpate the heartbeat of her child as her abdomen begins to swell? When a mother can synchronize her attention with that of her baby and then sense her own rate simultaneously, the vagus nerve (pacemaker of the heart and organizer of the social nervous system) develops optimally.

What is the instinctual biological dynamic being expressed and how can it be differentiated? How can it be held in its wholeness? Differentiation is not separation but rather a differentiated wholeness. Differentiated wholeness is an embodied wholeness. This is one role of therapeutic support assumed by anyone working with pregnant moms. It is important to differentiate the intake narrative of origin from communication with the infant as a spontaneous heart-felt emergence of intimacy. This is holding the whole. But remember, does mom feel comfortable talking to her baby? These therapeutic communications are rather basic/general qualities of presence and represent personal and professional training that would be necessary and essential to safely engage in that process with clients and their prenates/infants.

3. *Connect with Community.* This includes friends, family, and spiritual advisors. Find the friends that can hear *the story that needs to be told at that moment.* The emotional ups and downs of pregnancy can be journaled or blogged if sharing with a friend is not available.

In addition, is there someone in mom's life who she feels she has a spiritual connection with (whatever that term might mean to each individual)? How can the sacred and compassionate nature of pregnancy be supported, and by what practices: mindfulness meditation, acupuncture, pregnancy massage, homeopathy, and so forth? Practitioners supporting pregnant moms must hold the pregnancy as a *great act of compassion* and take that to heart, feel it empathetically in the heart, and be moved to act with gentleness and kindness for more effective therapeutic relationships with pregnant moms and families. Therapists must give the gift of fearlessness to pregnant moms.

4. *Connect with Professionals.* Do so when necessary to have questions answered and fear reduced. These practitioners include midwives, doulas, obstetricians, psychotherapists, and a whole host of other professionals who provide care to women and girls in the preconception, prenatal, and early parenting periods. Identifying feelings of safety with each professional is the crucial element of the relationship. Women trying to conceive and pregnant moms should seek out the professionals who generate a feeling of safety. Moms and professionals must mutually acknowledge feelings of a lack of safety and choose behaviors and actions that support safety and trust.

Cardioception (from the first step above) is a critical method of measuring safety inwardly and consciously. The key is to reduce fear in pregnant moms and families. As such, all professionals need to have exquisite listening skills for the many stories pregnant moms have to tell. Finally, as mentioned above, it is important to do follow-up with moms after a session of any kind. We are also advocating for resourcing of moms in between sessions so the whole pregnancy is supported. Compassion does not end when the client leaves the office.

References

Andreone, J., Lacoste, B., and Gu, C. (2015) 'Neuronal and vascular interactions.' *Annual Review of Neuroscience 38*, 25–46.

Birnholz, J., Stephens, J., and Faria, M. (1976) 'Fetal movement patterns: A possible means of defining neurologic developmental milestones in utero.' *American Journal of Roentgenology 150*, 537–540.

Boddy, A.M., Fortunato, A., Sayres, M.W., and Aktipis, A. (2015) 'Fetal microchimerism and maternal health: A review and evolutionary analysis of cooperation and conflict beyond the womb.' *Bioessays 37*, 1106–1137.

Brodsky, D., and Christou, H. (2004) 'Current concepts in intrauterine growth restriction.' *Journal of Intensive Care Medicine 19*, 1–13.

Buckley, S.J. (2015) *Hormonal Physiology of Childbearing: Evidence and Implications for Women, Babies and Maternity Care.* Washington, D.C.: Childbirth Connection, National Partnership for Women and Families. Available at www.nationalpartnership.org/research-library/maternal-health/hormonal-physiology-of-childbearing.pdf, accessed on 26 September 2016.

CDC (2016) *Tobacco Use and Pregnancy: How Does Smoking During Pregnancy Harm My Health and My Baby?* Available at www.cdc.gov/reproductivehealth/maternalinfanthealth/tobaccouse pregnancy, accessed on 26 September 2016.

Danese, A., and McEwen, B.S. (2012) 'Adverse childhood experiences, allostasis, allostatic load, and age-related disease.' *Physiology and Behavior 106*, 1, 29–39.

de la Cruz, M.V., and Markwald, R.R. (eds) (1998) *Living Morphogenesis of the Heart.* Boston, MA: Birkhauser.

Durand, E.F., Logan, C., and Carruth, A. (2007) 'Association of maternal obesity and childhood obesity: Implications for healthcare providers.' *Journal of Community Health Nursing 24*, 3, 167–176.

Gillman, M.W. (2008) 'Developmental Origins of Obesity.' In F.B. Hu (ed.) *Obesity Epidemiology.* New York: Oxford University Press.

Haig, D. (1993) 'Genetic conflicts in human pregnancy.' *Quarterly Review of Biology 68*, 4, 495–532.

Haig, D. (1996) 'Altercation of generations: Genetic conflicts of pregnancy.' *American Journal of Reproductive Immunology 35*, 3, 226–232.

Harvard T.H. Chan School of Public Health (2016) *Prenatal and Early Life Influences: Understanding Obesity's Developmental Origins.* Available at www.hsph.harvard.edu/obesity-prevention-source/obesity-causes/prenatal-postnatal-obesity, accessed on 26 September 2016.

Holt, S., and Patterson, N. (2006) *Ghost in Your Genes.* Boston, MA: Holt Productions, and BBC.

Hrdy, S.B. (1999) *Mother Nature: Maternal Instincts and How they Shape the Human Species.* New York: Ballantine.

Hunt, J. (2006) 'Stranger in a strange land.' *Immunological Reviews 213*, 36–47.

Huppertz, B., Burton, G., Cross, J., and Kingdom, J. (2006) 'Placental morphology: From molecule to mother – a dedication to Peter Kauffman – a review.' *Placenta 27, Supplement A, Trophoblast Research 20*, S3–S8.

Kallenbach, L.R., Johnson, K.L., and Bianchi, D.W. (2011) 'Fetal cell microchimerism and cancer: A nexus of reproduction, immunology, and tumor biology.' *Cancer Research 71*, 1, 8–13.

Karanam, V.L., Page, N.M., and Anim-Nyame, N. (2010) 'Hypoxia in pre-eclampsia: Cause or effect?' *Current Women's Health Reviews 6*, 1–6.

Kirby, M. (2007) *Cardiac Development.* New York: Oxford University Press.

Lanius, U.F. (2014) 'Dissociation and Endogenous Opioids: A Foundational Role.' In U.F. Lanius, S.L. Paulsen, and F.M. Corrigan (eds) *Neurobiology and Treatment of Traumatic Dissociation.* New York: Springer.

Lupien, S.J., McEwen, B.S., Gunnar, M.R., and Heim, C. (2009) 'Effects of stress throughout the lifespan on the brain, behaviour and cognition.' *Nature Reviews Neuroscience 10*, 6, 434–445.

Mahmood, U., and O'Donoghue, K. (2014) 'Microchimeric fetal cells play a role in maternal wound healing after pregnancy.' *Chimerism 5*, 2, 40–52.

Monk, C., Spicer, J., and Champagne, F.A. (2012) 'Linking prenatal maternal adversity to developmental outcomes in infants: The role of epigenetic pathways.' *Developmental Psychopathology 24*, 4, 1361–1376.

Myatt, L. (2006) 'Placental adaptive responses and fetal programming.' *The Journal of Physiology 572*, 1, 25–30.

Nathanielsz, P.W. (1996) *Life Before Birth: The Challenges of Fetal Development.* New York: Freeman.

Porges, S. (2004) 'Neuroception: A subconscious system for detecting threats and safety.' *Zero to Three.* Available at www.frzee.com/neuroception.pdf, accessed on 26 September 2016.

Rasanen, J., Wood, D.C., Debbs, R.H., Cohen, J., Weiner, S., and Huhta, J.C. (1998) 'Reactivity of the human fetal pulmonary circulation to maternal hyperoxygenation increases during the second half of pregnancy: A randomized study.' *Circulation 97*, 257–262.

Relier, J-P. (2001) 'Influence of maternal stress on fetal behavior and brain development.' *Biology of the Neonate 79*, 3–4, 168–171.

Rijnink, E.C., Penning, M.E., Wolterbeek, R., Wilhelmus, S., *et al.* (2015) 'Tissue microchimerism is increased during pregnancy: A human autopsy study.' *Molecular Human Reproduction 21*, 11, 857–864.

Saad, A., Dickerson, J., Gamble, P., Yin, H., *et al.* (2016) 'High fructose diet in pregnancy leads to fetal programming of hypertension, insulin resistance and obesity in adult offspring.' *American Journal of Obstetrics and Gynecology 215*, 3, 378, e1–6.

Sandman, C.A., and Davis, E.P. (2012) 'Neurobehavioral risk is associated with gestational exposure to stress hormones.' *Expert Review of Endocrinology and Metabolism 7*, 4, 445–459.

Scaer, R.C. (2007) *The Body Bears the Burden: Trauma, Dissociation and Disease* (2nd edition). New York: The Haworth Medical Press.

Scaer, R.C. (2012) *8 Keys to Brain-Body Balance.* New York: Norton.

Seng, J.S., Low, L.K., Sperlich, M., Ronis, D.L., and Liberzon, I. (2011) 'Post-traumatic stress disorder, child abuse history, birthweight and gestational age: A prospective cohort study.' *BJOG 118*, 11, 1329–1339.

Shonkoff, J.P., Boyce, W.T., and McEwen, B.S. (2009) 'Neuroscience, molecular biology, and the childhood roots of health disparities: Building a new framework for health promotion and disease prevention.' *JAMA 301*, 21, 2252–2259.

Sibley, C.P., Turner, M.A., Cetin, I., Ayuk, P., *et al.* (2005) 'Placental phenotypes of intrauterine growth.' *Pediatric Research 58*, 5, 827–832.

Simeon, D., Giesbrecht, T., Knutelska, M., Smith, R.J., and Smith, L.M. (2009) 'Alexithymia, absorption, and cognitive failures in depersonalization disorder: A comparison to posttraumatic stress disorder and healthy volunteers.' *The Journal of Nervous and Mental Disease 197*, 492–498.

Szejer, M. (2005) *Talking to Babies: Healing with Words on a Maternity Ward.* Boston, MA: Beacon Press.

Thomson, P. (2007) '"Down will come baby": Prenatal stress, primitive defenses and gestational dysregulation.' *Journal of Trauma and Dissociation 8*, 3, 85–113.

Tomanek, R.J., and Runyan, R.B. (eds) (2001) *Formation of the Heart and its Regulation.* Boston, MA: Birkhauser.

Van den Bergh, B.R., and Marcoen, A. (2004) 'High antenatal maternal anxiety is related to ADHD symptoms, externalizing problems, and anxiety in 8- and 9-year-olds.' *Child Development 75*, 4, 1085–1097.

Van den Bergh, B.R., Mulder, E., Mennes, M., and Glover, V. (2005) 'Antenatal maternal anxiety and stress and the neurobehavioral development of the fetus and child: Links and possible mechanisms. A review.' *Neuroscience and Biobehavioral Reviews 29*, 237–258.

Wadhwa, P.D. (2005) 'Psychoneuroendocrine processes in human pregnancy influence fetal development and health.' *Psychoneuroendocrinology 30*, 724–743.

Wadhwa, P.D., Culhane, J.F., Rauh, V., Barve, S.S., *et al.* (2001) 'Stress, infection and preterm birth: A biobehavioral perspective.' *Paediatric Perinatal Epidemiology 15*, Suppl. 2, 17–29.

Wadhwa, P.D., Entringer, S., Buss, C., and Lu, M.C. (2011) 'The contribution of maternal stress to preterm birth: Issues and considerations.' *Clinical Perinatology 38*, 3, 351–384.

Wadhwa, P.D., Glynn, L., Hobel, C., Garite, T., *et al.* (2002) 'Behavioral perinatology: Biobehavioral processes in human fetal development.' *Regulatory Peptides 108*, 149–157.

Weinstein, A.D. (2016) *Prenatal Development and Parents' Lived Experiences: How Early Events Shape our Psychophysiology and Relationships.* New York: Norton.

Whitaker, R.C. (2004) 'Predicting preschooler obesity at birth: The role of maternal obesity in early pregnancy.' *Pediatrics 114*, 29–36.

Yehuda, R., Engel, S.M., Brand, S.R., Seckl, J., Marcus, S.M., and Berkowitz, G.S. (2005) 'Transgenerational effects of posttraumatic stress disorder in babies of mothers exposed to the World Trade Center attacks during pregnancy.' *Journal of Clinical Endocrinology Metabolism 90*, 7, 4115–4118.

CHAPTER 2

THE EFFECTS OF MATERNAL TRAUMA ON CHILDREN'S PSYCHOLOGICAL HEALTH

Professor Franz Ruppert

Trying to understand the human psyche is a highly complex issue (Ruppert 2012a). The deeper we delve into the psyche the more we understand how it develops during life, and how it develops coping strategies (or not) in response to life's challenges, threats and insults.

Social interaction between individuals has a special significance for humans because we are designed to exist and survive in social groups. To be part of these, to get material support, to be really seen, to be understood emotionally, and to be respected as a person, we have to open ourselves up to others. We feel with them and we suffer if they suffer. Perhaps we even sacrifice aspects of ourselves, our egos, for that connection and support.

The mother–child bond

Because we develop in a womb environment, the relationship to one's own mother is extraordinarily important. There is a very special and unique psychological and emotional bond between mother and child. This is no new scientific discovery; this awareness is part of our everyday experience. Observing emotionally healthy mothers watching intensely over their children, and children clinging onto their mothers with all their might, reveals the unique and incomparable bond between a mother and her child.

John Bowlby and Mary Ainsworth

Not until the middle of the last century did psychology, psychiatry and psychotherapy really explore the topic of the mother–child bond. The British psychoanalyst John Bowlby (1907–1990) had to combat the doctrines of psychoanalysis to defend his concept of attachment against the predominant view which argued that it was mostly sexual and aggressive instincts that form our basic make-up and determine our character. Bowlby insisted that a child doesn't love his mother just because she feeds him. He identified a child's need for closeness and body contact with his mother as the very intrinsic need of every newborn (Bowlby 1973, 1998).

Bowlby and his colleagues proved in experimental trials that there is a specific attachment behavior in children which is always activated when they lose contact with their mothers. Children run after their mothers, call them and cry so that their mothers come back into contact. In situations of danger or stress they will seek contact with their mothers. The mother is their 'emotional safe base' with whom they can release stress and feel safe enough to allow their attention to be drawn outwards to their surroundings. One of John Bowlby's colleagues, Mary S. Ainsworth (1913–1999), also showed that mothers have different mechanisms to manage their children's stress. She differentiated three kinds of mother–child bond (Ainsworth 1973):

- *Secure attachment:* In a secure attachment, physical contact with a mother can calm a child, his stress hormone levels fall and after a while he will feel calm and content again.

- *Ambivalent-insecure attachment:* In an ambivalent-insecure attachment it is significantly more difficult to soothe a stressed child. Part of him may even resist physical contact with his mother. He cries for longer and hormonal stress levels don't return completely to normal. The child's conflict is whether his mother is a source of stress rather than a resource for stress release. (Ways of working with this type of behavior are discussed in Chapter 11.)

- *Avoidant-insecure attachment:* In an avoidant-insecure attachment, experiencing the mother as a source of stress is considerably enhanced. The child can't release stress even when in contact with his mother. He still needs contact with his mother, yet after frustrating experiences in trying to bond he keeps his distance and often waits passively. Observers perceive him as withdrawn and sulky; his behavior is self-contained.

Research has also shown that secure attachment encourages a child's orientation towards his surroundings. Trusting that his mother is always a secure support and source of comfort, the child explores his environment fearlessly, plays with more interest and makes contact with other children more easily (Bowlby 2001). A secure attachment therefore encourages the development and sense of autonomy. Ambivalent-insecure children on the other hand tend to be more attached and 'clingy', as exemplified in difficulties getting them to bed in the evening. In normal, healthy development, from the age of three, a securely bonded child can withstand his mother's increasingly prolonged absences because he has a clear, stable, anchored sense of her within his own psychological make-up. However, if he has experienced difficulties in having his needs met by his mother, as part of the normal symbiotic mother–child bonding, then *he is much less able* to detach psychologically from her at various other age-appropriate phases as he progresses through childhood and into adult life, and this can cause immense suffering and distress.

Current attachment research

Research into attachment has become more refined recently and increasingly enables more precise insights into the nature of early childhood attachment. I would refer the reader to the publications of Karin and Klaus Grossmann (2004) and Karl Heinz Brisch (2013, 2014) which summarize the current position of attachment theory and research. Thanks to improved investigation methods it is possible to conclude with certainty that, amongst other things:

- the bond between mother and child develops during pregnancy and that the child in the womb is very sensitive to his mother's moods and feelings (Zimmer 1998)

- the birth process and the support the mother gets from experienced women such as doulas has a significant influence on whether a mother embraces her baby lovingly or whether she sees her baby as the cause of pain (Klaus, Kennell and Klaus 2002)

- the first hour after birth is a highly sensitive phase for establishing attachment between mother and child (Klaus and Klaus 1999)

- the quality of attachment between mother and child is different from that between a father and his child (Grossmann *et al.* 2002).

Because of the fundamental importance of the mother–child bond for a person's healthy development, nature tries to protect it at all costs. The behavior of a mother and her child naturally fit together like a lock and key. This is why during pregnancy, birth and postnatally mothers need the support of other women, especially those who themselves have undergone the experiences of pregnancy, birth and motherhood. Unfortunately, the prevailing medical disease model of pregnancy and birth can undermine the development of a secure attachment between mother and child and promote fear and stress instead of joy (Zandl 2003; Ruppert 2014). For example, if Caesareans are performed electively rather than in situations of medical necessity, it can disrupt highly sensitive developmental processes under the diktat of medical risk and financial considerations. This obviously has ramifications for babies, families and society as a whole if the end result is children becoming more dysfunctional or hyperactive.

The mother–child bond from the perspective of psychotrauma theory

My research model for a deeper understanding of the human psyche is my own practical work as a psychotherapist. I owe deep insights into the functioning of the human psyche to a particular method which I developed (Ruppert 2012b, 2014). My therapeutic work validates the fundamental theories of human development formulated by John Bowlby, namely that the mother–child bond constitutes the 'internal working model' for all emotionally important attachments later in life. Simply put, in therapy work one can observe these tendencies:

- In the adult choice of partners, a subconscious selection process tends to err towards those who recapitulate frustrated maternal attachment patterns.

- Needs that were not met by their mother are acted out in attachment styles with their own children.

- Early mother–child conflict patterns are repeated in workplace conflicts with superiors and colleagues.

- The closer and more intensive the attachment to another person gets, the more those early patterns of the original mother–child bond are recapitulated. That is also true in friendships and relationships between a therapist and his clients.

Conversely, this also means that a secure mother–child bond becomes a fundamental resource for attachment structures later in life. A person who has a mother anchored as a stable ground for support, warmth, comfort, understanding, trust and love doesn't have to marry a person full of fear, self-doubt and mistrust. Furthermore, he doesn't have to entangle others in his own emotional problems; he knows how to regulate his emotions and where his own responsibilities begin and end. He can trust his own strengths. He has a healthy ego which can connect with other healthy egos and can establish boundaries to protect himself from others who don't.

Fortunately, the nature of the mother–child bond is often so resilient that it survives even the unconscious behavior of mothers and young children in a society dominated by consumerism and commercialism. Educational styles have only a negligible influence on the quality of the mother–child bond; and in my therapeutic experience I found that the most sustained influences on this are traumatic experiences in a mother's life. On the basis of my long-term work with many mentally ill people I would like to suggest that lasting attachment disorders that are difficult to heal in the mother–child bond develop only if the mother had traumatic experiences in her own life.

Psychotrauma

To explain this thesis, we need a general definition of what is generally understood by 'psychotrauma'. In their textbook on psychotraumatology, Gottfried Fischer and Peter Riedesser define traumatic experiences as 'a vital experience of discrepancy between threatening situational factors and the individual's potential to cope with them, accompanied by feelings of helplessness and defenselessness which causes a lasting disruption of their self- and world-view' (Fischer and Riedesser 2003, p.79).[1] My definition

---

1   Text originally in German.

would expand this further to include the concept that our coping strategies for dealing with stress not only fail to protect us, but they even enhance the threatening situation and then have to be inhibited by other unconscious survival strategies. This happens through rigidifying of movements, freezing of feelings, dissociating of thoughts and the splitting up of the personality into three different psychological parts (Figure 2.1):

- healthy parts

- traumatized parts

- trauma-survival strategies.

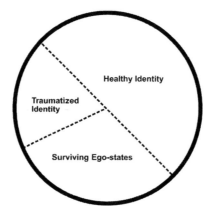

Figure 2.1 Fracturing of the human psyche after a traumatic experience

In scientific literature the definition of trauma is often limited to that of 'shock' and the experience of existential impotence or powerlessness. Since the basis of the human psyche is not merely the desire to survive but also the need for relationship, I suggest classifying traumatic experiences into four categories:

- existential trauma

- the trauma of loss

- attachment trauma or the 'trauma of love'

- attachment system trauma.

'Existential trauma' is all about life and death. It is about physical survival in a situation such as a natural disaster or a survived attempted abortion.

In this case the main perception is the fear of death. Despite surviving such a situation, increased levels of tension and fear can remain which might manifest later in life with symptoms such as repeated panic attacks.

In a 'trauma of loss' a person loses an important attachment figure as a result of death or due to a person's constant emotional or physical absence (e.g. if a child's mother is dissociated, mentally ill or dies early). Fears of being abandoned, anger, pain and grief are the feelings that can remain after an experience of traumatic loss. Long-term effects might be chronic depression.

In a 'trauma of love' the need for attachment itself is traumatized. This means that the child's attempts to bond with his mother are hopeless because she evades her child's every emotional approach or overwhelms him with her own trauma patterns. The more the child seeks emotional closeness, the greater the emotional distance the mother creates between herself and her child in order to protect herself from being overwhelmed by her own repressed trauma. Fear of being alone, anger, despair and even self-hatred can be engendered in a child caught in an attachment trauma situation. The most difficult aspect for the baby or child is the subjugation of his own identity in order to adapt to the mother's coping strategies. Since the mother is not able to be in touch with healthy aspects of her ego, it makes it very hard for the child to do the same.

The 'trauma of love' therefore becomes the means whereby traumatized attachments extend into entire 'attachment systems' (i.e. whole families). Because such adults do not have the capability or awareness to take responsibility for what they do or don't do, there is the potential for things to happen in families which fundamentally contradict the nature of a mother–child bond. In extreme cases a mother might kill her own child or there is parental abuse. This can result in children attaching themselves to an offending mother in a highly confused emotional way. Psychotic and schizophrenic conditions are the long-term results of such family dynamics often associated with violence between men and women and between parents and their own children. In such an attachment system anyone can be either a perpetrator or a victim and as a rule ends up being both concurrently (Ruppert 2012b).

Trauma does not disappear by itself. Even if psychological traumas are suppressed they continue to affect the subconscious. Triggered by situations similar to the original trauma, the ability to suppress them often no longer works, and the person in question experiences re-traumatization.

However, because the memory of original trauma is suppressed, the person doesn't always know the source of these associated overwhelming feelings. He might feel himself out of control or feel that he doesn't understand himself any more.

Attachment and trauma

In attachment research, attention is increasingly focusing on the close relationship between attachment and trauma (Hesse and Main 1999; Brisch 2003; Schechter 2003; Ruppert 2014). Traumas can massively compromise the mother–child bond from early on:

- If the conception is already a traumatizing experience for the woman (e.g. in the case of abuse or rape), it is going to be difficult to welcome her child into life with love.

- Any abuse or violence against a woman during the pregnancy will also traumatize the child.

- Women who have experienced existential traumas can be overanxious and have a tendency to be over-protective of their children. They might strictly control their children and give them little space to develop at their own pace and in their own way. They can even impose their own fear of death on their children.

- Women who have experienced a loss trauma can be overwhelmed by feelings of pain and grief when they see and feel their newborn baby. On the other hand, the baby might perceive pain and a deep sadness in his mother's eyes. Pain and sadness become the basis of his own perception of her. It is difficult for him to dissociate from his mother and he often ends up becoming a mother substitute for his own mother.

- Women who have experienced attachment traumas can pass their fear, anger and despair onto their own children. On the one hand they expect the kind of affection from their children which they themselves did not receive from their own mothers, whilst on the other hand they reject the child in the same way that they were rejected by their own mothers. If they experienced sexual abuse, there is also the potential that they will not be able to protect their own children from it and even bring them unwittingly into situations where the child is exposed to similar dangers.

- Women who grew up in families which hid behavior that contradicts the basic principles of attachment often pass their own confused feelings on to their children. These children can then have real problems in perceiving clear feelings and in differentiating what feels right or wrong. This can fundamentally undermine the development of a child's own identity.

Consequences for children if a mother is traumatized

A psychologically healthy mother is a great resource for a child and a blessing for his entire life. Conversely, traumatized mothers can be a heavy burden for their children:

- A child can feel completely abandoned even in the womb if he cannot feel his mother. This might be because she is emotionally numb in her abdomen as a result of some sexual violence, for example.

- Traumatized mothers may be unable to sense their bodies and therefore nourish themselves inadequately or wrongly. They might even smoke or drink alcohol as trauma survival strategies, which harms the unborn child directly.

- It is also possible that the unborn witnesses conflicts between his mother and his father, which puts him under stress.

- If a traumatized mother does not empathize enough with him during the birthing process, the child can find himself in an existential emergency situation before and during birth which might be so unbearable that he has to split apart psychologically.

- If the newborn baby doesn't encounter an emotionally present mother after birth because she is sedated with anesthesia and painkillers or perhaps dissociated, this also can create a situation of excessive demand and helplessness. He can only survive with a further separation of his feelings, his own needs, and finally his own ego.

- Since traumatized mothers are often with men who are also highly traumatized, they cannot sufficiently protect their children from neglect and violence. The children have to give up a lot of themselves and finally even their own sense of self to be able to go on living in such environments.

- Traumatized mothers can have distorted perceptions around the real needs of their babies: they are fed, but what they are actually seeking is closeness and body contact. They might be left alone much too long, or left in the hands of inappropriate people. These children eventually switch off altogether and then might seem especially easy to care for because they essentially give up and no longer cry or protest.

The significance of the father bond

Over-emphasizing the significance of the mother–child bond for our mental health leaves us wide open to criticism from two sides. First from mothers who might feel that they are solely responsible if their children's development goes awry, and second from fathers who don't feel validated in their role in bringing up their children. I intend neither. The fact that a child's emotional attachment to his mother is by nature completely different and substantially more emotional and intense than the attachment to his father does not mean that fathers don't contribute anything essential to their children's psychological foundations. Ideally, the love fathers have for their partners can enhance and support a woman's love for their children. The support men give their partners also supports their children, too. A father's love gives additional psychological strength to his son or daughter and offers a male perspective on their world. The child needs his father differently than his mother. A father can't replace the mother bond, in the same way that a mother can't replace the father's role for the child (Garstick 2013).

Identity-oriented psychotraumatherapy

The quality of the mother–child bond is, to a certain extent, pre-programmed by the traumas in a woman's life. Her trauma experiences are mirrored in her children. This is a frightening fact because we can foresee that a woman who has experienced an attachment trauma is likely to pass on her negative attachment experiences to her child. The child in need of attachment looks for support in his mother but he has to split himself apart to attach to his mother. He binds part of himself to his mother's survival part and another part to his mother's traumatized part. And in so doing he subsumes the maternal trauma into his own psychological make-up. In this way psychological traumas are passed on from generation to generation.

In the past I hesitated to recommend therapies to pregnant women. Nowadays I think we urgently need to inform pregnant women about how their attachment experiences from their own early years will be re-stimulated by contact with their children from the very beginning.

Having a child does not solve these problems. If a young woman feels empty and alone on the inside and she hopes that she will be able to break out of this inner hollowness by having her own child, she is mistaken. The sooner a mother is supported in understanding her own psychological problems and in solving them, the better the attachment to her child will be. Psychological help is often too late if the attachment between mother and child is already severely disrupted. Counseling and specific therapies aimed at the mother–child bond can achieve a lot more than intervention measures which merely scratch the surface, such as approaches that only focus on a child's behavioral disorders. There is no sense in treating a hyperactive child without realizing that this child has probably absorbed feelings of fear, anger and restlessness from his mother and may be traumatized by the attachment to her.

Dealing with attachment disorders related to one's mother tends to be the central focus in most adults' therapies. To overcome the 'trauma of love' a person has to work through a lot of resistance and survival strategies because a child will always try to love his traumatized mother with all his might. A person can only successfully detach himself from his mother if the very traumatizations which arose from the attachment to a traumatized mother in the first place are seen and felt. To do that in therapy, the healthy ego has to come to the fore and be supported. Only then can the confrontation with the trauma be endured in the here and now. I developed a method especially suited for groups which I call *Selbstbegegnung mit dem Anliegensatz*, which roughly translated means 'meeting yourself through stating your intention'. First, the client formulates his issue to be addressed and writes it down in a sentence for all the others to see. Then he chooses a person from the group for each of the words in this sentence of intention. These individuals sense into resonance with each particular word. In this way the client explores his inner make-up, his ego, his will, his feelings, and so on, and he can develop the single components of his psyche further in order to heal the whole.

Conclusion

In summary, if we look at how attachment impacts society as a whole, this means that everything that helps a mother to offer a secure emotional attachment to her child is to be welcomed. Whatever benefits are given to mothers by a social community benefits society as a whole.

References

Ainsworth, M. (1973) 'The Development of Infant–Mother Attachment.' In B.M. Caldwell and H.N. Ricciuti (eds) *Review of Child Development Research* (Vol. 3). Chicago: University of Chicago Press.
Antonovsky, A. (1997) *Salutogenese – zur Entmystifizierung der Gesundheit.* Tübingen: dgvt-Verlag.
Berndt, C. (2015) *Resilienz. Das Geheimnis der psychischen Widerstandskraft.* München: dtv-Verlag.
Bowlby, J. (1973) *Attachment and Loss (Vol. II). Separation: Anxiety and Anger.* New York: Basic Books.
Bowlby, J. (1998) *Attachment and Loss (Vol. III). Loss: Sadness and Depression.* London: Random House.
Bowlby, J. (2001) *Das Glück und die Trauer.* Stuttgart: Klett-Cotta. (*The Making and Breaking of the Affectional Bonds.* London: Tavistock Publications, Chapters 1–7; and *International Review of Psychoanalysis,* Chapter 8.)
Brisch, K.H. (1999) 'Familiäre Bindungen. Die transgenerationale Weitergabe familiären Bindungsverhaltens.' In *Psychoanalyse der Familie.* Gießen: Psychosozial-Verlag.
Brisch, K.H. (2003) 'Bindungsstörungen und Trauma.' In K.H. Brisch und T. Hellbrügge (Hg.) *Bindung und Trauma.* Stuttgart: Klett-Cotta Verlag.
Brisch, K.H. (2013) *Schwangerschaft und Geburt.* Stuttgart: Klett-Cotta Verlag.
Brisch, K.H. (2014) *Säuglings- und Kleinkindalter.* Stuttgart: Klett-Cotta Verlag.
Fischer, G., and Riedesser, P. (2003) *Lehrbuch der Psychotraumatologie.* München: Reinhardt Verlag.
Garstick, E. (2013) *Junge Väter in seelischen Krisen.* Stuttgart: Klett-Cotta Verlag.
Grossmann, K., and Grossmann, K.E. (2004) *Bindungen – das Gefüge psychischer Sicherheit.* Stuttgart: Klett-Cotta Verlag.
Grossmann, K., Grossmann, K.E., Fremmer-Bombik, E., Kindler, H., and Scheuerer-Englisch, H. (2002) 'The uniqueness of the child–father attachment relationship: Fathers' sensitive and challenging play as a pivotal variable in a 16-year longitudinal study.' *Social Development 11,* 3, 301–337.
Hesse, E., and Main, M. (1999) 'Second-generation effects of unresolved trauma in non-maltreating parents: Dissociated, frightened, and threatening parental behaviour.' *Psychoanalytic Inquiry 19,* 481–540.
Klaus, M.H., and Klaus, P.H. (1999) *Your Amazing Newborn.* Cambridge, MA: Perseus.
Klaus, M.H., Kennell, J., and Klaus, P.H. (2002) *The Doula Book.* Cambridge, MA: Perseus.
Ruppert, F. (2012a) *Symbiosis and Autonomy.* Steyning: Green Balloon Books.
Ruppert, F. (2012b) *Trauma, Angst und Liebe.* München: Kösel Verlag.
Ruppert, F. (2014) *Frühes Trauma. Schwangerschaft, Geburt und erste Lebensjahre.* Stuttgart: Klett-Cotta Verlag.

Schechter, D.S. (2003) 'Gewaltbedingte Traumata in der Generationenfolge.' In K.H. Brisch und T. Hellbrügge (Hg.) *Bindung und Trauma.* Stuttgart: Klett-Cotta Verlag.
Zandl, M. (2003) *Lukas. Erkenntnisse einer Mutter.* Neumünster: Edition Taufpatenclub.de.
Zimmer, K. (1998) *Erste Gefühle. Das frühe Band zwischen Kind und Eltern.* München: Kösel Verlag.

Further information

Further information on attachment and trauma can be found at www.franz-ruppert.de.

CHAPTER 3

POLYVAGAL THEORY AND VAGAL TONE IN BABIES

Dr Carolyn Goh

The nervous system is perhaps the most complex and important circuit in the human body. It is made up mainly of the central nervous system and the peripheral nervous system. The autonomic nervous system (ANS) is part of the peripheral nervous system and is also known as the involuntary nervous system. It regulates the functions of internal organs such as the stomach and heart and operates below the level of our consciousness. Some of the other functions of the ANS are to regulate heart rate, blood pressure and digestion.

Historically, the ANS was described as having two opposing components: the parasympathetic nervous system (PNS) and the sympathetic nervous system (SNS). The SNS is known as the 'quick response mobilizing system'. It exhibits the classic fight-or-flight response to a perceived harmful event, attack or threat to survival. The body goes into a state of heightened awareness such as dilation of the pupils and vasoconstriction occurs to direct blood to vital organs and muscles. There is an increase in blood pressure, heart rate and muscle tension. In this state, less energy is available for other functions such as digestion of food and repair of the body. Long-term heightened sympathetic activity can have detrimental effects on health in the long term as the body's immune system is suppressed, making it more vulnerable to infection (Carlson 2013).

The parasympathetic nervous system is known as the 'rest, digest and heal system'. Some of its functions are to control salivation, lacrimation, urination, defecation and digestion. One very important component of the PNS is the tenth cranial nerve called the vagus nerve. Vagus is Latin for 'wandering', and it is an accurate description of this nerve. The vagus nerve emerges at the back of the skull, makes its way through the abdomen, and branches out to the heart, lungs, voicebox, stomach and ears, among other body parts (Berthoud and Neuhuber 2000). It is responsible for bringing the body back into homeostasis (balance) after activation of the SNS.

Stephen Porges

In 1994, Dr Stephen Porges discovered that the two-part model of the ANS was not a true depiction of the nervous system. During his research on the vagal nerve in babies, Porges discovered that in fact there are two different vagus circuits, making a total of three ANS circuits. The two circuits come from two different areas of the brain stem, and they evolved sequentially, one far earlier than the other (Porges 2007). This led him to develop what is known as the Polyvagal Theory.

These vagal systems have evolved from an unmyelinated vagus nerve in reptilians to a myelinated vagus circuit in humans. Mammals have two vagal circuits, one potentially lethal, and the other protective: the reptilian parasympathetic, unmyelinated vagus nerve and the 'social engagement' myelinated vagus nerve (Porges 2009).

The reptilian vagus system is characterized by immobilization or freezing. Reptiles play dead or freeze when under attack. The mammalian nervous system developed to incorporate the sympathetic fight-or-flight response in order for mammals to run away or fight off predators and a social engagement nervous system that makes full use of face-to-face interaction to evaluate how safe a situation is.

These systems are all imbedded in our physiology in a hierarchical order. For example, if a rat senses danger, being a mammal its first line of action is the fight-or-flight response. If, however, it is still under threat and unable to escape, it resorts to the older reptilian nervous system of immobilization. It faints.

Humans use the social engagement system to assess the safety of a situation. This involves reading facial expressions, listening to speech and voice, and assessing other behaviours in fellow humans. If we feel uncomfortable or less safe, we then engage the fight-or-flight response (sympathetic nervous system) to escape from the situation. If, however, we are unable to flee or escape the situation, we resort to the reptilian nervous system of immobilization; in other words, we freeze.

Immobilization due to fear can have detrimental and sometimes lethal consequences. A mouse that is recovering after a trauma that caused immobilization will die soon after the trauma (Porges 2004). Humans will likely start to develop acute stress symptoms if the nervous system is not 're-set'. These stress symptoms correspond to the vagal circuit being turned off, resulting in reduced parasympathetic activity such as digestive problems and an inability to sleep. Porges suggests that people who suffer repeated anxiety attacks throughout their lives may well be under the influence of repeated vagal reflex immobilizations as their nervous system has not been re-set post-trauma (Porges 2004).

The vagus in the baby

Prenatal babies, newborns, small infants and young children are most susceptible to trauma as their intelligence, emotional regulation and perceptional systems are underdeveloped. The absence of safe adults, insecure boundaries, and exposure to threat and danger overwhelm them. Their nervous systems go into shutdown and freeze. Later, as the infant enters puberty and young adulthood, inaccurate neuroception often becomes more 'hardwired', and the child may respond inappropriately to life situations (Porges 2004).

The myelinated vagus circuits (the social engagement system) in humans provide more rapid and tightly organized responses linked to brain stem areas that regulate the muscles of the face and head (Porges 2009). This circuit influences our middle-ear muscles by changing our capacity to hear predators or low-frequency sounds (Lamb, Freund and Lerner 2010). In a safe environment, the vagal circuit is working and the middle-ear muscles dampen the surrounding low-frequency sounds, allowing the person to pick up on sounds such as the human voice. When there is something in the environment that threatens us, we turn off the vagal circuit as it gets in the way of moving to fight or flight (Lamb *et al.* 2010). This pattern of events is seen often in autistic children (Porges 2004).

Hearing and responding

An interesting aspect of the Polyvagal Theory is the subject of 'hyperacusis', whereby the neuroception detects sound frequencies which indicate threat but processes them to a much more sensitive degree, shifting the nervous system into fight-or-flight mode (Porges *et al.* 2014). Hyperacusis is likely to be a major explanation for the often random and sometimes aggressive behaviours that autistic children can exhibit (Porges 2004).

Humans interpret low-frequency sounds as predatory. A person with a shut-down vagal system is more alert to the low-frequency sounds due to the changes in the middle-ear muscle (Lamb *et al.* 2010). This becomes very significant when we look at therapy or treatment environments. If the treatment room is noisy, with sounds from traffic and ventilation systems, the client's physiology is going to be in a hypervigilant defence mode (Porges 2004). This is especially true when dealing with clients who are children or babies or who have experienced trauma. In order to come out of the hypervigilant mode, the body must recognize that it is safe. Once our senses (sight, hearing, etc.) evaluate the situation is safe, the signal is sent through the myelinated vagus nerve that inhibits the fight-or-flight response and the body calms down.

The nervous system in a healthy individual is able to re-engage the social engagement system fairly quickly, taking the person out of fight-or-flight mode once the body feels safe. However, if a person has experienced a traumatic experience causing immobilization, it is more difficult to re-set the nervous system. Music therapy (Porges 2008), meditation and breathing exercises such as pranayama yoga can be used to stimulate vagal activity.

A baby will listen out for his or her mother's voice, the smell of his mother and familiar faces. These are vagal triggers that can trigger the vagus nerve and soothe a hypervigilant baby. It is important to remember that babies take longer to respond to these signals as their vagal tone is not fully developed. At birth, babies do not have a fully developed nervous system. They exhibit a lower vagal tone, which increases as they develop (Field and Diego 2008).

Studies by Porges and colleagues (Doussard-Roosevelt *et al.* 1997) show that the vagal tone in babies is reduced below three months of age, and in some babies right up till six months of age. This has a profound effect on how the nervous system responds to situations and stimuli. When vagal tone is low, this means that the ability of the nervous system to 'correct' itself when it goes out of balance is hampered. A useful analogy is the brakes of a car. Dampened vagal reactivity can be likened to the car's brakes that have gone 'soft'. The car takes a long time to respond to the braking action (inhibit fight-or-flight) and continues on its path before gradually slowing down. In babies, the fight-or-flight response is not inhibited and the body stays in a state of heightened tension and anxiety for some time.

So, a baby with low vagal tone will easily get stuck in a state of tension and anxiety when they experience a stressful situation. The baby will be difficult to settle, have sleep problems and may also experience digestive problems. This is similar to what adults experience in times of stress: symptoms such as heartburn, indigestion, anxiety and insomnia. Therapies such as Bowen (Wilks and Knight 2014), craniosacral therapy and massage (Diego *et al.* 2007; Field and Diego 2008) are thought to have a beneficial effect on helping the nervous system develop by stimulating vagal activity. Social face-to-face interaction is also an important factor in engaging the social feedback system and stimulating vagal activity (Field and Diego 2008). Therapists can use their skills of social engagement by using appropriate prosody, facial expression and slowing their movements down to encourage positive vagal tone.

A mature and well-developed vagal tone allows the nervous system to fluctuate between states of heightened sympathetic activity in times of stress and return to the calmness of the parasympathetic state. Research (Dockray 2014; Perez-Burgos *et al.* 2013) into the microbiome population of the infant gut and the role it plays in the development of the vagus nerve and the gut brain axis is also shedding new light on the importance of gut flora, birthing methods, breastfeeding and nutrition.

References

Berthoud, H.R., and Neuhuber, W.L. (2000) 'Functional and chemical anatomy of the afferent vagal system.' *Auton. Neurosci. 85*, 1–3, 1–17.

Carlson, N. (2013) *Physiology of Behavior.* New York: Pearson.

Diego, M.A., Field, T., Hernandez-Reif, M., Deeds, O., Ascencio, A., and Begert, G. (2007) 'Preterm infant massage elicits consistent increases in vagal activity and gastric motility that are associated with greater weight gain.' *Acta Paediatr. 96*, 11, 1588–1591.

Dockray, G.J. (2014) 'Gastrointestinal hormones and the dialogue between gut and brain.' *J. Physiol. 592*, Pt 14, 2927–2941.

Doussard-Roosevelt, J., Porges, S.W., Scanlon, J., Alemi, B., and Scanlon, K. (1997) 'Vagal regulation of heart rate in the prediction of developmental outcome for very low birth weight preterm infants.' *Child Development 68*, 173–186.

Field, T., and Diego, M. (2008) 'Vagal activity, early growth and emotional development.' *Infant Behav. Dev. 31*, 3, 361–373.

Lamb, M.E., Freund, A.M., and Lerner, R.M. (2010) *The Handbook of Life-Span Development: Social and Emotional Development.* Hoboken, NJ: Wiley.

Perez-Burgos, A., Wang, B., Mao, Y.K., Mistry, B., *et al.* (2013) 'Psychoactive bacteria Lactobacillus rhamnosus (JB-1) elicits rapid frequency facilitation in vagal afferents.' *Am. J. Physiol. Gastrointest. Liver Physiol. 304*, 2, G211–G20.

Porges, S.W. (2004) 'Neuroception: A subconscious system for detecting threats and safety.' *Zero to Three 24*, 5, 19–24.

Porges, S.W. (2007) 'The polyvagal perspective.' *Biol. Psychol. 74*, 2, 116–143.

Porges, S.W. (2008) *Music Therapy & Trauma: Insights from the Polyvagal Theory.* Symposium on Music Therapy & Trauma: Bridging Theory and Clinical Practice. New York: Satchnote Press.

Porges, S.W. (2009) 'The polyvagal theory: New insights into adaptive reactions of the autonomic nervous system.' *Cleve. Clin. J. Med. 76*, Suppl. 2, S86–S90.

Porges, S.W., Bashenova, O., Bal, E., Carlson, N., *et al.* (2014) 'Reducing auditory hypersensitivities in autistic spectrum disorder: Preliminary findings evaluating the Listening Project protocol.' *Front. Pediatr. 2*, 80.

Wilks, J., and Knight, I. (2014) *Using the Bowen Technique to Address Complex and Common Conditions.* London: Singing Dragon.

CHAPTER 4

ATTACHMENT, BRAINS AND BABIES

HOW WE ARE SHAPED BY OUR
EARLIEST RELATIONSHIPS

Graham Kennedy

Introduction

The human baby, when compared with the young of all other mammals, is incredibly vulnerable and totally dependent on others meeting its needs. This vulnerability is in part an evolutionary trade-off. Human babies, and the babies of other primates, have a much larger brain in relation to body size than the young of all other mammals. Human adults also have a much smaller pelvis than our evolutionary ancestors as a result of us walking upright on two legs. The combination of these two factors means that the human baby has to be born at a much earlier stage of his or her developmental process in order to be able to pass safely through the mother's pelvis. If human babies were born at the same developmental stage as other animals, we would need to have a gestational period of approximately 18 months, and give birth to a baby the size of a nine-month-old.

As a consequence of this, human babies are unable to care for themselves and to meet their own primary needs. Because they require the longest period of care, protection and nurturing of any species, there needs to be a way in which their primary caregivers[1] feel motivated enough to expend the time, energy and effort required to look after them. How, then, does the

---

1   I use the term primary caregiver as opposed to parents to highlight the fact that it is not only the infant's biological parents that can be the primary attachment figures. Adoptive parents, foster parents, grandparents, kinship carers and even childminders, nannies and teachers can also be primary attachment figures.

vulnerable newborn baby ensure his survival? He does this through the development of highly specialized attachment-based behaviours that have significant impacts on the brains of both the baby and his primary caregivers, and develops a bond that endures for life.

The attachment process is not only of critical importance in helping a baby develop a strong loving relationship with his caregivers, it also becomes the model for all our future relationships. The nature of our early attachment relationship also has significant effects on our psychological, emotional, social, behavioural and educational development.

Most people will be much more familiar with the term 'bonding' than they are with attachment. Both of these terms have been used extensively and often interchangeably for several decades to describe the way in which the intimate relationship between a baby and his primary caregivers develops. Before going further, I think it is important to define these terms and to understand the differences between them.

A bond is a special relationship which we have with important others in our life. We have a bond with our families, with our children, with friends, with people that we share interests and experiences with. We can even have a bond with our pets. However, a bond is very different from an attachment relationship. An attachment relationship is a specific type of bond that develops through infancy and early childhood between the infant and his primary caregivers (most commonly his biological parents), and has four defining characteristics.

The first characteristic is that the caregiver acts as a safe haven to which the infant can return in times of need or distress. The second characteristic is that the caregiver is a secure base from which the infant can begin to move out and explore the world. The third is proximity seeking, where infants insist on staying close to their caregivers in times of stress or distress. The fourth is separation distress, where the infant becomes distressed when separated from their caregiver.

From these definitions, it becomes clear that attachment is something that infants do to their primary caregivers, and not the other way around. For example, a parent doesn't turn to her child for safety and support, but rather to her partner, friends and family. In the attachment literature, caregivers are often described as having affectional bonds with their children, whereas children have an attachment relationship with their caregivers.

The early history of attachment theory

Over the past 60 years, attachment theory has influenced a wide spectrum of society, including the hospital care of children, adoption and fostering policy, and day-care policies. However, the main area that has been affected has been in the understanding of the importance of the relationship between a baby/child and his primary caregiver.

Attachment theory began with the work of John Bowlby and Mary Ainsworth. In the 1950s, Bowlby, a British psychoanalyst, undertook a detailed study for the World Health Organization on the mental health effects that hospitalization and institutionalization had upon children. At that time, hospital visits from parents were actively discouraged, and limited to one hour per week. This rigid protocol was set in place, amongst other reasons, as a result of the belief that parents could easily contaminate their sick child with germs from the outside world.

Bowlby found that the effects of maternal deprivation on children in hospital were similar to those he observed in institutionalized children. These effects included lack of empathy, inability to give and receive affection, aggression, violence and depression. This led him to conclude that what babies and young children need for optimum well-being is a warm, intimate and continuous relationship with their mother, or an appropriate substitute. As a result of these experiences, and from his private practice at the Tavistock Clinic in London, Bowlby began to formulate the basis of what was to become his theory of attachment.

Mary Ainsworth, a developmental psychologist, worked with Bowlby at the Tavistock Clinic in the 1950s. In 1954, she left the clinic to undertake research on the interactions between mothers and their babies in Uganda. This research set her on the path to the realization that it is the quality of parenting and the responsiveness of the primary caregiver towards her baby that are instrumental in creating specific styles of attachment.

As a result of her detailed research, Ainsworth was able to categorize different styles of attachment based on her now famous Strange Situation experiments, in which babies between the ages of nine and 18 months are separated from their primary caregiver for a short period of time, and then reunited. What is important about this is not just how the babies respond to the separation, but more crucially how they respond to their caregiver on reunion.

From these experiments, Ainsworth was able to classify a secure style of attachment and two types of insecure attachment: avoidant and ambivalent. The later work of Mary Main defined a fourth attachment style: disorganized. The securely attached babies were able to explore and play freely in the presence of their caregiver, were visibly upset when they left the room, and were readily comforted on their return. Ainsworth described this type of attachment as ideal, and both she and many subsequent researchers have observed that around two-thirds to three-quarters of all children have a secure attachment.

The insecurely attached infants responded in markedly different ways to both separation and reunion, compared with those who were securely attached. Avoidantly attached infants will play with toys in the presence of a caregiver, but are unlikely to involve the caregiver in the play. On separation, they are unlikely to be distressed, and tend to ignore or move away from their caregiver on their return. Avoidantly attached children tend towards being overly self-reliant and independent, and tend to avoid both closeness and intimacy.

Ambivalently attached infants are unable to use their caregivers as a secure base for exploration, and tend to stay close, and even cling to them even before there is separation. They are highly distressed on separation and not easily soothed on reunion. Children with ambivalent attachment tend towards insecurity, clinginess and an over-reliance on their caregivers.

The infants who have a secure, avoidant or ambivalent style of attachment each have an organized strategy for dealing with separation and distress. However, the final category of infants has no such sense of internal organization, and tends to respond to distress in an unpredictable, contradictory or even chaotic way. These are the infants that have a disorganized attachment. As children, their behaviour is often chaotic and unpredictable. They have difficulty trusting people, and often have an innate need to control everyone and everything in their environment.

In the years since Bowlby's and Ainsworth's initial findings, there has been an explosion of research into attachment, with particular emphasis on the neuroscience of how these early formative relationships impact a baby's developing brain.

Babies' brains

Our brains have three main functional areas: the brainstem (reptilian brain), the social and emotional limbic system (mammalian brain) and the neocortex (rational brain). The reptilian brain is the oldest, most primitive part of our brain and is responsible for instinctive behaviour related to safety and survival. It is the only part of the brain that is fully operational at birth. The other two parts of the brain develop postnatally.

Jaak Panksepp, a leading neuroscientist, has shown that the reptilian brains of all mammals contain seven genetically ingrained emotional centres[2] that are intimately associated with the attachment process (Panksepp and Biven 2007). Three of these, the Fear, Rage and Separation Distress/Panic centres, are frequently triggered in babies and young children, giving rise to states of emotional distress and dysregulation.

Babies and young children are totally dependent on the more mature regulatory capacities of their caregivers to help calm these episodes of distress, which usually manifest as intensive crying episodes and tantrums. This is due to the fact that the higher regulatory centres in their brains are not yet fully developed. If these dysregulated states are not regularly and appropriately attended to by a sensitive caregiver, then these emotional states can ultimately become ingrained personality traits, creating lifelong patterns of rage, fear and panic in emotionally stressful and anxiety-provoking circumstances.

The development of three of the other emotional systems in the brain, the Play, Care and Seeking systems, is also dependent on the regulation of these more primitive dysregulated states. Without the development of emotional regulation, these three systems may not fully develop, leading to deficiencies in our ability to play, to nurture others and to explore our environment.

So how is it that these regulatory behaviours are able to calm and soothe a dysregulated baby? In the brain, it is the right hemisphere that is primarily involved in the processing of social-emotional information, and it is particularly sensitive to facial expressions, tone of voice and other non-verbal information coming from caregivers.

The prefrontal cortex (PFC), located just behind the forehead, is responsible for many of our higher functions that differentiate us from other

---

2   These seven emotional systems are Rage, Fear, Separation Distress/Panic, Care, Seeking, Play and Lust (which is not developed in children).

mammals and primates. These include social-emotional development and the ability to regulate our emotional impulses, both of which are important components in the development of attachment security. As with the right hemisphere, the PFC is highly sensitive to the attuned non-verbal responses of the primary caregiver, and even depends on them for its maturation and development.

To understand this further, we need to look at the work of Stephen Porges, a leading authority on the autonomic nervous system (ANS). He has updated the old model of a two-tier ANS to include a third aspect, the social engagement system, which is mediated by the ventral vagus nerve. He also coined the term neuroception to describe how we are constantly subconsciously monitoring our environment to assess it for safety and threat (Porges 2011).

The ventral vagus is also particularly sensitive to the non-verbal aspects of communication in relationships. Porges has shown that when there is a neuroception of safety, and the ventral vagus is activated through such interactions as appropriate eye contact, tone of voice and facial expressions, it has the capacity to over-ride and subdue the more defensive sympathetic and parasympathetic responses of fight, flight and freeze, which are characteristic of more dysregulated states.

It is these everyday non-verbal, face-to-face interactions which take place many times a day between primary caregiver and baby that develop the social and emotional (mammalian) aspect of the baby's brain, and in which the essence of the attachment relationship is developed. It is for this reason that attachment researchers tend to focus on parenting styles as the primary factor involved in the development of attachment security.

Secure attachment

Attachment researchers have shown that attachment security is most effectively developed through regular and consistent interactions that emphasize both attunement and affect regulation. Attunement requires that the primary caregiver is sensitive to the needs and other signals of the infant. An important aspect of attunement is the sharing of affective states so that the caregiver is able to match the rhythm and intensity of the other's experience.

So, for example, if an infant is upset, the caregiver can respond in an attuned way by modulating their tone of voice, facial expressions, gestures and other non-verbal communication to match the level of affect in the infant, without needing to directly experience the emotion of the upset themselves. This, as Dan Siegel (1999) describes, allows the infant to feel 'felt' by their caregiver, an essential component of attachement.

Dan Hughes, a leading researcher and clinician in the field of attachment therapy, describes how an attuned response needs to have four main qualities for it to be effective. These qualities are Playfulness, Acceptance, Curiosity and Empathy (PACE), and together constitute his Dyadic Developmental Psychotherapy (DDP) model of working with attachment issues.

Playfulness involves a lightness of interaction, a sense of mutual engagement and enjoyment of each other's company, as well as utilizing positive affective states such as joy, humour and laughter. Acceptance is about accepting the inner world and reality of the child without necessarily condoning the behaviour. For example, a baby or young child, who in a moment of intense frustration throws his plate of food on the floor, needs to be met with an acceptance of his frustration and need to throw his food in that moment. This is in direct contrast to a more punitive approach that focuses on the 'wrongness' of the behaviour, which creates a sense of shame and leads to mis-attunement.

It is worth noting at this point that many parents believe they need to be 'getting it right' in a fully attuned way at least 80–90 per cent of the time for their baby to develop a secure attachment. Fortunately for all us imperfect parents, research shows that attachment security can develop when caregivers are fully attuned a third of the time, they are somewhat attuned a third of the time, and they are completely mis-attuned a third of the time. This is somewhat reassuring as no-one can correctly interpret, or be in a place to accurately meet, the needs of their children all of the time.

In fact, it is an essential part of the attachment process that caregivers do not get it right all of the time. For secure attachment to develop, babies and young children need to experience frequent ruptures in the attachment relationship. However, what is critical about these ruptures is not whether they happen or not, as in all relationships this is a given, but how effective is the repair in the form of comforting and re-attuning that follows. This relational repair also needs to contain the four qualities of PACE.

The third component, curiosity, is an attitude of not-knowing, but a willingness to try to understand what is really going on for a child, as opposed to making guesses or assumptions based on their behaviour. The final quality, empathy, is an essential component of all healthy relationships. It is the capacity to know, and directly relate to, the difficult experiences of another person. Unfortunately, rather than meet a child with empathy, we are often too quick to criticize, to give advice and to try to fix whatever 'difficulty' they are presenting us with. For the child, empathy from his caregivers creates a sense of being understood and acknowledged for exactly how they are. It also serves as a useful model by which the child can begin to develop his own empathy towards others.

An example of attunement can be seen when a young child and his caregiver play a normal game of peek-a-boo. In this game, the adult and child are sitting opposite each other where they can observe each other's faces. The caregiver begins the game by slowly lifting a towel up to hide her face from her child. As she does this, the child begins to giggle with anticipation of what comes next. In response to this, the caregiver lowers the towel slowly in order to heighten her child's level of anticipation. The child begins to giggle even more, until at the last moment the caregiver reveals her whole face as she goes 'boo'. Both caregiver and child begin laughing together, each enjoying the interaction with the other. During this whole process, both caregiver and child are intensely focused on each other. Each one is actively helping to modulate both the tempo and the anticipation level of the game by being firmly attuned to the other person.

As with attunement, affect regulation is also an integral part in the development of attachment security. In fact, so much so that Allan Schore, a leading researcher in this field, has described the attachment process as primarily a regulatory process (Schore 1999). A newborn baby, although much more sentient and aware than was previously believed, is nonetheless unable to regulate his own states of emotional distress, and is totally dependent on his primary caregiver being able to do this for him.

Insecure attachment

If good attunement and affect regulation lead to secure attachment, it would make sense that those infants who have developed patterns of insecure attachment have experienced differing degrees of mis-attunement and a lack of appropriate regulation. It would also make sense that the stresses of these mis-attuned and dysregulating experiences would have a negative effect on the developing brain. This is exactly what the research on parenting styles shows.

Unfortunately, many caregivers have unresolved emotional issues arising from their own early life that can get in the way of them responding appropriately and sensitively. For example, a mother who is insecure and unsupported in her parenting role may be unable to accurately and appropriately meet the needs of her baby. Similarly, a father who never received the nurturing and comfort he needed as a baby and young child may be insensitive to the similar needs in his own child.

Approaches to parenting are also socially and culturally driven. For example, in the UK, there is a tendency to down-play healthy emotional development at the expense of intellectual or athletic achievement. This is reflected in such phrases as 'pull yourself together', 'just get on with it' and 'put a lid on it', which reflect a basic lack of awareness of our emotional needs.

Avoidantly attached infants tend to have primary caregivers who are emotionally unavailable and insensitive to their emotional needs. This emotional unavailability comes from the fact that they themselves received a similar type of parenting when they were children, and as a result they are often dismissive of the importance of true emotional intimacy in their relationships with partners and with their children. Because avoidantly attached adults tend to parent in a way that creates avoidant attachment in their children, we can see that this creates a style of attachment that is perpetuated through the generations.

Children with ambivalent attachment have been found to have primary caregivers who were inconsistent and unreliable in terms of their emotional availability and attunement. In some instances they were able to meet the child's needs, and in others they were either absent or overly intrusive. Consequently, the child is left feeling uncertain as to whether their needs will be met or not at any given time. These caregivers tend to be overly preoccupied with events and perceived injustices that occurred to them when they were children. As a result, these children tend to be overly clingy, dependent and needy in terms of their relationships with parents, teachers and, later on, partners.

Where levels of caregiver mis-attunement and dysregulation become severe, the infant is at high risk of traumatization and developing disorganized attachment. The primary caregivers of these infants have been found to have high levels of their own unresolved trauma, loss or fear in relation to their own attachment history. As a result, they are unable to effectively regulate themselves, let alone meet the needs of their infants. They are also unable to provide a secure enough base for the infant, as they are a primary source of terror and dysregulation. As a result, these children are caught in the paradox of needing to be comforted when distressed, but the person they need to be comforted by is also the source of that distress.

Trauma and attachment

Whilst the type of parenting that a child receives is the primary organizer of their attachment style, it is not the only one. The effects of traumatic experiences can also take their toll on our capacity to relate to others.

However, when talking about attachment, not all traumas are equal. Because attachment is a relational process that develops through infancy and early childhood, the most severe forms of trauma are those perpetrated in these early months and years by our primary caregivers, who are supposed to be sources of safety and security. These relational traumas, such as neglect and abuse, involve a massive failure in both attunement and emotional regulation by the primary caregiver. In fact, he/she is responsible for inducing extreme levels of stimulation and arousal in their child: extremely high levels in the case of abuse, and extremely low levels in the case of neglect.

Whilst the traumas inflicted on children through abuse and neglect are horrific, it is the absence of a safe, secure adult that really causes the damage. What can make all the difference to these children is having one person in their lives who can act as a secure base; someone who has the capacity for both attunement and emotional regulation. This person can be a grandparent, a neighbour, a teacher or even a therapist. By being a consistent presence in a child's life, they help to mitigate the most damaging effects of these horrific traumas.

Abuse and neglect are also not the only forms of trauma that can impact attachment, although they are the most severe. High levels of prenatal stress and trauma, for example from excessive cigarette and alcohol consumption, maternal rejection, attempted abortion, drug use and domestic violence, can adversely affect the developing brain of the foetus. This is discussed elsewhere in this book.

Other traumatic incidents that can impact on an infant's attachment style include prematurity, postnatal depression, early hospitalizations and invasive hospital procedures, bereavement, and separation from, or loss of, a primary caregiver.

Highly stressed and traumatized babies often develop behaviours such as inconsolable crying or parental rejection (pushing their caregivers away) that require even more sensitive parenting and understanding than their non-stressed counterparts. As a result of this behaviour, and the caregivers' subsequent frustration, sleeplessness and feelings of being overwhelmed, it can be particularly challenging for them to accurately attune to their baby's needs, and to help regulate their particularly high levels of emotional arousal.

These caregivers often find they need significant extra support to help them meet the needs of their infants. However, if they are able to find the support they need (whether from friends, family or therapeutic support), and are able to meet their infant's needs, then this can dramatically influence the development of the infant's attachment style, regardless of the nature of the trauma experienced. This shows that it is the relational experience as opposed to the actual traumatic incident that is the determining factor as to how a child's attachment security is adversely affected.

Effect on brain development

Relational traumas such as abuse, neglect, separation and loss cause significant damage to the child's developing brain. High levels of cortisol and other stress hormones have a toxic effect on synaptic development, an essential process for brain maturity. These children also have over-active Fear, Rage and Separation Distress/Panic systems, which can lead to significant behavioural and psychological problems.

If we look at what is happening in the brain in terms of Porges's polyvagal system, these children are not receiving the socially attuned interactions they need to regulate their constant state of distress and alarm. As a result, there is a constant neuroception of threat, and the ventral vagus is no longer effective in inhibiting the more primitive defensive responses of the ANS. Instead, the sympathetic nervous system and the dorsal vagus generate the conditions of fight, flight and freeze, which further reduces the child's capacity for prosocial engagement.

These children find it incredibly hard to regulate their emotional responses. As a result, they commonly display disruptive behaviours combined with dissociation and impairments in attention and cognition. They also display compromised coping and social skills, tendencies to violence, and are vulnerable to developing psychiatric disorders such as post-traumatic stress disorder.

Attachment and adoption

One group of children for whom an understanding of attachment and early trauma is particularly important are those that have been adopted. There was a time when the majority of adopted children were babies who had been relinquished by mothers who felt unable or unwilling to look after them. Today, very few babies are relinquished. Instead, the majority of babies and children who enter the care system do so because they have been removed from their birth families by social services.

There has also been another change in adoption demographics in that today very few babies, outside of sibling groups, are placed for adoption. In fact, the average age for a child in the UK to be adopted is 3–4 years old. It is also a sobering fact that three-quarters of those children who are adopted have been removed from their families as a result of some kind of abuse or neglect. As well as this, there is often a history of parental drug and alcohol abuse, mental illness and domestic violence.

As a consequence, many adopted children have to deal with the effects of multiple traumas and separations. These not only include the traumas experienced while living with their birth family, but also being removed from their birth parents, and possibly from their siblings as well. Once removed they are placed into foster care, and can commonly move foster homes several times before an adoptive family is found. This constant movement from house to house, school to school and family to family is a frightening, disorienting and bewildering experience. Most importantly, it adds to the feelings of loss and separation, and also prevents the formation of a stable attachment with a primary caregiver.

Many of these children often go on to develop a variety of emotional and behavioural problems affecting just about every area of their lives. These include difficulties in forming close relationships, extreme hypervigilance, difficulties with change and transition, aggressiveness, oppositional defiance, developmental problems and learning difficulties, as well as emotional issues due to their unresolved grief, rage and shame.

Many adoptive parents find that they are suddenly presented with a child who does not conform to the norms of their world, to their outlook on life and to their values. They also find that this child does not respond to normal methods of parenting and often requires more specific, therapeutic approaches.

What they are told, however, time and again by friends, family and social workers, is that all these children need is a secure, loving home and that over time they will begin to settle and adapt to their new, more functional lives. However, not only is this not true, it sets parents up to fail and feel like failures. When they have their child placed with them, adoptive parents will try to create a safe and secure environment in which they can begin the process of bonding and attachment to their child. This is a normal, healthy response to the arrival of a new child in a family. However, it is this very sense of safety, security and closeness that many of these children have a problem with.

Children whose brains have been hardwired by abuse, neglect, chaos and unpredictability feel deeply threatened by the love, security and closeness that a healthy, functional family offers. They often respond by trying to control those around them or going into a more primitive fight, flight or freeze response.

This creates conflict, confusion and increased stress in the parents. On the one hand, they are doing everything right for their child, but he still wants to lash out, scream at them, run away or attack them. What commonly happens is that the chaos and stress of the child's birth family gets re-created in their adoptive family as a result of the child's challenging behaviour. Parents frequently get burnt out, relationships start to suffer and break down, and one or both parents can start to suffer from depression and the symptoms of vicarious trauma.

Attachment and the therapeutic relationship

One of the positive findings that has come from attachment research is that, even if a child did not develop a secure attachment with their primary caregivers, it is never too late. In the right conditions, we can develop what is known as an earned security even once the formative window of infancy and early childhood has closed. One of the main ways in which this can be achieved is through working with a therapist who has a good understanding of attachment dynamics.

Therapeutic work with both adults and children who have suffered disrupted attachment needs to be multi-faceted. It needs to address any unresolved emotional issues associated with them not getting their attachment needs met. It needs to create a coherent narrative to help them make sense of their experiences. It may also need to address the effects of specific traumas, and help regulate a dysregulated nervous system.

There are a number of treatment approaches that can help to achieve this. In some cases, it may be possible to find a practitioner who is able to cover all of these bases, but if not, a multidisciplinary approach may be the most effective way forward. Since attachment is primarily a relational process, it is those therapies that emphasize the relational nature of the work that tend to be the most effective in helping to develop earned security. These are most typically the talking therapies, for example counselling and psychotherapy, especially where the qualities of PACE are an integral part of the work. Other therapeutic approaches such as craniosacral therapy and homeopathy can also play their part.

The therapist takes the role of a primary caregiver, providing a safe haven and secure base for the client to explore their own attachment history. It is also essential that the therapist is able to maintain their own emotional regulation and to act as a model of secure attachment for their client.

When it comes to working with children, and especially those who have experienced high levels of trauma and disruption, there are a number of factors that need to be taken into account.[3] First, they require a much more specialized approach, as normal talking therapies are often ineffective with these children. One of the reasons for this is that many of these children have adopted pathological lying as a survival strategy and, as is often the case, if they are seen on a one-to-one basis without the involvement of the primary caregivers, the child can easily run rings around an unsuspecting therapist. I know of several cases where this has led to a child making untrue allegations of abuse to the therapist against a parent.

Another reason why some approaches can be ineffective is that they are primarily non-directive. This means that the therapist is not directly interfering with, or influencing, the direction that the session takes. Instead, they adapt

---

3   When it comes to adopted children, the current law in the UK states that only those therapists who are part of an Ofsted-registered Adoption Support Agency can offer therapeutic support.

and respond to whatever the client chooses to discuss. One of the challenges of this is that traumatized children will rarely if ever spontaneously disclose difficult aspects of their life story, and their associated feelings.

What these children need are approaches to therapy that encompass both directive and non-directive methods, and also give the child an opportunity to explore the more difficult aspects of their history in a safe and non-threatening way. If possible, it is also recommended that the primary caregivers be included in the therapy sessions, as repairing any disruption that has taken place in their relationship will be a major focus of the sessions.

There are a number of therapies whose effectiveness in working with children with extreme levels of disrupted attachment has been clearly demonstrated. These include Dan Hughes's DDP, art therapy, Theraplay, music therapy, drama therapy, equine therapy and filial therapy. Integrative approaches that combine different aspects of these therapies can also be very effective.

Other approaches, such as craniosacral therapy and homeopathy, as well as occupational therapy support to work on any unresolved sensory issues, may also help to support the therapeutic process. It may also be important for the child's primary caregivers to get support in terms of therapeutic parenting strategies to help them deal more effectively with any behavioural problems that they might be struggling with.

References

Panksepp, J. and Biven, L. (2007) *The Archaeology of Mind: Neural Origins of Human Emotion* (1st edition). New York: Norton.

Porges, S.W. (2011) *The Polyvagal Theory: Neurophysiological Foundations of Emotions, Attachment, Communication, and Self-Regulation.* New York: Norton.

Schore, A.N. (1999) *Affect Regulation and the Origin of the Self: The Neurobiology of Emotional Development.* Hillsdale, NJ: Lawrence Erlbaum.

Siegel, D.J. (1999) *The Developing Mind: Towards a Neurobiology of Interpersonal Experience.* New York: Guilford Publications.

Further reading

Ainsworth, M., Blehar, M., Waters, E., and Wall, S. (1978) *Patterns of Attachment: A Psychological Study of the Strange Situation.* Hillsdale, NJ: Lawrence Erlbaum.

Bowlby, J. (1969) *Attachment and Loss (Vol. I): Attachment.* Harmondsworth: Penguin.

Hesse, E. and Main, M. (2000) 'Disorganized infant, child, and adult attachment: Collapse in behavioral and attentional strategies.' *Journal of the American Psychoanalytic Association 48*, 4, 1097–1127.

Hughes, D.A. (2009) *Attachment-Focused Parenting: Effective Strategies to Care for Children.* New York: Norton.

Perry, B. (2014) *The Effects of Trauma and Neglect on Childhood Development.* Adoption UK Conference talk, 15 November. Available at www.adoptionuk.org/sites/default/files/documents/ BondingAttachment1.pdf, accessed on 23 January 2017.

Schore, A.N. (2001a) 'Effects of a secure attachment relationship on right brain development, affect regulation, and infant mental health.' *Infant Mental Health Journal 22,* 1–2, 7–66.

Schore, A.N. (2001b) 'The effects of early relational trauma on right brain development, affect regulation and infant mental health.' *Infant Mental Health Journal 22,* 1–2, 201–269.

Sunderland, M. (2007) *What Every Parent Needs to Know: The Incredible Effects of Love, Nurture and Play on Your Child's Development.* London: Dorling Kindersley.

CHAPTER 5

EVERY BABY HAS A STORY TO TELL

MEMORY CRYING AND BABY BODY LANGUAGE AS AN EXPRESSION OF EXPERIENCE IN BABIES

Matthew Appleton

The emerging field of pre- and perinatal psychology

The general consensus amongst medical practitioners and scientists is that babies do not experience pain at birth and retain no memory of the experience. This is based on an understanding of neurological development and the nature of memory that is rapidly becoming outdated. At odds with this prevailing understanding is the clinical experience of practitioners in a number of different therapeutic disciplines, who have encountered birth and prenatal memories in their work with clients. This includes dream recall and associated imagery in psychoanalysis (Rank 1929; Fodor 1949; Share 1994), the medical use of LSD (Lake 1966; Grof 1976), breathing techniques (Grof and Grof 2010), hypnosis (Gabriel and Gabriel 1995; Chamberlain 2013), spontaneous regressions during bodywork (Upledger 1990) and specific embodied birth and prenatal simulation techniques (Emerson 2000).

Over the past 50 years or so many thousands of people have participated in workshops which have facilitated prenatal and birth regression processes. Drawing from this experience, researchers have mapped out how various prenatal and birth events are embodied and how these are accompanied by specific body language. For example, the psychiatrist R.D. Laing recounts a female client talking about her husband wanting a divorce: 'It was a body blow right here (pointing to the navel)' (Laing 1976, p.73). This 'body memory' of the earlier trauma of the premature cutting of the umbilical cord and separation from the mother was stimulated by the present-moment trauma of her husband's intention to separate.

The stages of birth

William Emerson, a pioneer in the emerging field of pre- and perinatal psychology, delineated four stages of birth from the baby's perspective, constellating around existential and psychological themes, with associated physiological consequences (Emerson 2004a). In brief, Stage 1 corresponds to the baby descending into the pelvic inlet and meeting the closed cervix. The themes of 'beginnings' and 'no-exit' are associated with this stage. Stage 2 relates to the rotation of the baby's head in the mid-pelvis. Themes associated with this stage are 'trust' and 'orientation'. Stage 3 is about moving through the pelvic outlet. 'Exhaustion' and 'being seen' are the major themes. Stage 4 begins with the birth of the head and body, through to the time that a family settles without any external interference from medical staff. The themes of 'exposure', 'separation' and 'invasion' belong to this stage. Unresolved trauma from any of these stages often shows up in later life, usually at times of transition such as going to school for the first time, moving home, coming in and out of relationship, even leaving the house.

When any of these stages becomes activated in the present moment, either through regression in a therapeutic setting or by a present-moment event that stimulates the 'body memory', specific body language associated with that stage is unconsciously activated. Each of these stages has 'conjunct sites' and 'conjunct pathways' associated with them. A conjunct site is an area of the body, usually the cranium, that was compressed by an area of the maternal pelvis during the birth process. A conjunct pathway is a pathway of compression left from being pushed over a maternal pelvic bone by contractions during labour. When the old birth trauma is activated, the person's hands unconsciously touch these conjunct sites and move along the conjunct pathways. When working in a clinical session with a baby, these types of hand movements are seen again and again. An example of this would be if a Stage 3 trauma was being activated, then the hands draw down over the face, mimicking the movement of the foetal face passing along the curve of the sacrum. In sessions with adults this might be accompanied by feelings of exhaustion and statements like 'I just can't go on' or 'I just keep hitting this brick wall'. If the umbilical cord was compressed by contractions during this stage, there may be accompanying feelings of panic and the sense that 'I can't breathe'.

Larimore and Farrant (1995) describe seven body movements associated with the early cellular processes of sperm, ovum and the implantation of the blastocyst. Further mapping out of these very early territories and the associated body language were developed by other researchers, in particular William Emerson and Karlton Terry (Emerson 2004b; Terry 2005). That these early cellular experiences could have a resonance within our psyches and that specific cellular movements might be expressed at the level of the adult organism often evokes incredulity. The basis for this claim is the consistent revelation of these deeply human formative processes in therapy sessions and workshops, in the form of unconscious body language and associated imagery and emotions. These are images and body movements that would be hard to identify without a deep knowledge of human embryology, and the emotions echo existential and psychological themes that repeatedly show up in relation to specific embryological stages. They therefore represent a profoundly important stage of human experience that is not recognized by western psychology or medicine and is not honoured within western culture as significant.[1] The science that supports these therapeutic insights is slowly beginning to emerge. Evidence that consciousness is not simply an epiphenomenon of the brain but resides both at a cellular level in the tissues, and even as a field phenomenon, is amassing at the borders of the prevailing mechanistic paradigm (Chamberlain 2013).

Baby Body Language

The body language associated with prenatal and birth experience is known simply as 'Baby Body Language' (BBL) (Terry 2009). Whilst it is present throughout life, BBL tends to be diminished by an educational focus on cognitive, rather than expressive, concerns, along with punitive or inappropriate environmental responses to what is being expressed. Babies are as yet free of such inhibitions and so 'tell their stories' through their BBL in a very expressive and articulate manner. However, it is generally

---

1   This is not the case in many indigenous cultures, where conception, prenatal life and birth are seen as fundamental in the shaping of the individual psyche and well-being of society as a whole.

not recognized as such, and so not responded to with the awareness and empathy that enable the story to be 'heard'. Consequently, babies are left with their 'stories' trapped in their bodies and psyches and are alone in that experience. This is extremely distressing for babies, which they may express through inconsolable crying, fractious behaviour and disturbed sleep. Later in childhood these unheard stories turn up in nightmares or are played out in games. They give rise to anxieties, phobias, compulsive behaviour and violent outbursts (Share 1994).

With the knowledge gathered through decades of regressive work with adults, a few practitioners began working directly with babies (Emerson 2000; Terry 2009). BBL is universal, and every baby to a lesser or greater degree tells the story of their journey coming into the world through these movements. Karlton Terry, a pioneer in the understanding of BBL, describes these movements as being 'non-volition, non-random movements' (Terry 2009). They are non-volitional in the sense that they spontaneously arise out of body sensation, rather than as acts of conscious intention. For example, if I am thirsty the conscious intention arises within me to pour water into a glass and drink from it. If I touch an area of my head because a birth memory is being stimulated, it is a spontaneous gesture arising out of my unconscious. I may not even be aware that I am doing it. Yet it communicates something of my experience. In the same way, babies are not motivated by a conscious intention to convey their experience. Yet they do so from their experience of what is happening in their bodies. In this regard BBL is 'non-random'. It conveys meaning even though it is not motivated by the conscious intention to do so.

BBL can be differentiated from other spontaneous movements, such as those by which babies slowly develop their capacity to coordinate. There is usually an emotional component to BBL. Babies express distress or frustration as they touch various conjunct sites and pathways or enact early prenatal themes. There is an intensity and frequency to BBL that is quite distinct from other movements they make. Parents, especially mothers, will often *feel* that their babies are trying to communicate something that they are not 'getting'. Perhaps one of the greatest obstacles to acknowledging the presence of BBL, as a meaningful communication of experience, *is that it is so obvious!* How can a form of human expression that is so universal not have been recognized before now? It is like the fable of 'The Emperor's New Clothes' but in reverse. Instead of the exclaiming there is nothing there, when everyone is agreeing there is, we are saying there is something there, when the general consensus is that there is not. Students who train in working with BBL often say, 'How could I not have seen this before?' It is a revelation even to midwives, paediatricians, craniosacral therapists or osteopaths, who work regularly with babies. Perhaps the deeper question is, how can a theory (i.e. babies are insensible to their prenatal and birth experience) be so powerful that it blinds us to what is right before our eyes?

Pressures during birth

The non-volitional, non-random movements are the more active component of BBL. The conjunct sites and pathways are the 'fixed' components. These compressive forces and stress patterns become held in the connective tissues of the body (Upledger 1990). Indentations from maternal pelvic bones of the cervix can often be clearly seen on babies' craniums. The most obvious fixed BBL is the 'birth lie-side' (Terry 2009). This is the side of the baby that was against the mother's spine during the last few weeks of pregnancy and during labour. Although there are variations on the theme, most babies are in a transverse position in relation to the maternal pelvis during the last few weeks of the pregnancy. The head leads the descent into the pelvis (cephalic presentation), and as the baby descends, the neck flexes so that the baby's crown comes into contact with the cervix. During the descent the baby's head turns about 45 per cent so that it is now in an oblique position, usually with the baby's occiput facing either to the left or right anterior aspect of the maternal pelvis. In obstetric terminology these are known respectively as 'left occiput anterior' (LOA) and 'right occiput anterior' (ROA). The most common and effective presentation for moving through the average maternal pelvis is LOA. Other presentations might include occiput posterior (OP) (often described as 'back to back') and breech.

As babies descend into the pelvis, and especially with the onset of contractions, the lie-side of the cranium is compressed against a large mass of bone known as the lumbo-sacral promontory (LSP). This consists of the lower lumbar vertebrae and the superior aspect of the sacrum. As the labour proceeds, the baby's head and shoulders are pushed over the LSP. There will already be some compression in the lie-side from the tight squeeze within the womb during the last few weeks of the pregnancy. This is exacerbated during the birth as the foetal skull distorts to accommodate the pressure from the LSP. Although the neonate skull has the capacity to remould after birth, the stronger compressive forces remain held in the tissues. The lie-side can be identified by a number of different indicators. The cranium is generally more compressed on this side, with the eye closer to the midline and slightly inferior to the eye on the other side. This is due to the dragging forces exerted on the cranium as contractions push the baby over the LSP. As most babies rotate into the lie-side during the rotational stage of birth, the nose deviates away from the lie-side, due to pressure from the sacrum exerted on the nose as the baby turns into it. The shoulder on the lie-side is usually more contracted and the baby may tend towards a 'banana' shape mirroring the curve of the mother's lumbar spine.

As such we can say that the lie-side tends to hold the most intense aspects of the birth story. This is especially true of the connective tissues, which adapt to stress and hold the memory of any intense or traumatic experience (Upledger 1996). Gentle stimulation (through touch or even simply moving towards making contact) of conjunct sites and pathways usually elicits an emotional response, and babies will spontaneously re-enact aspects of their birth experience, especially the places where they became stuck (Peirsman and Peirsman 2006; Agustoni 2013). There tends to be more active BBL on the lie-side, with babies repeatedly touching the most prominent conjunct sites and pathways. Movements on the lie-side tend to be more jerky, as peripheral nerves may be compressed and more 'shock' is held on this side of the body. The emotional expression in the lie-side eye is often different than the non-lie-side eye. It may be less present or hold more fear or anger.

Memory crying

BBL is often accompanied by memory crying. This can be differentiated from a 'present-moment needs cry'. A present-moment needs cry is crying elicited by a present-moment issue that needs attending to, such as hunger, dehydration, discomfort due to heat or cold, boredom, tiredness, overstimulation or a soiled nappy. Most people are familiar with these forms of crying and are able to attend to them. Memory crying occurs when the memory of an earlier traumatic event surfaces. There are various theories of how memory becomes holographically imprinted at a cellular and tissue level (Pearshall 1988; Ho 1998; Oschman 2000; Barrett 2013; Verny 2014). In adults, birth and prenatal memories may surface as if they were holographically unfolding in the present. Images and emotions associated with the earlier event are experienced as a 'gestalt'. Being able to experience the intensity of the event, whilst retaining a conscious witness to it, enables an integration of the event at a higher level of consciousness, rather than have it operate unconsciously at the level of a threat to survival.

The memory crying of babies is clearly experienced as present-moment lived experience. BBL becomes more frequent, sometimes even frantic. The emotional expression which can be seen in the eyes and heard in the tone of crying alerts us to the existential theme that the baby is in contact with. Memory crying conveys one of three essential emotions: anger/rage, sadness/grief or anxiety/terror. Babies may look lost, alone, confused, pressured or withdrawn. These nuances interface with one or more of these three essential emotional qualities, giving us more clues as to what the crying conveys of their experience.

Insofar as memory crying is recognized for what it is and responded to appropriately, it can lead to a release of tension. If it is mistaken for a present-moment needs cry and is responded to with attempts to feed or pacify, either by 'shushing' or the use of a pacifier, it only leads to greater tension and distress. This can lead to cycles of ongoing distress for both the baby and the parents. From the parents' perspective they are trying to do everything they can to soothe their baby, but nothing works. This, in turn, leads to a loss of confidence, increased stress and frustration, often accompanied by exhaustion due to loss of sleep and tension between parents, as they both struggle with their own tension and tiredness. For the baby, who acutely feels the stress levels of the parents, this increases distress and tension, so that both baby and parents become trapped in a vicious circle of negative feedback, in which everyone feels isolated within their own sense of helplessness.

Parents may know that their child is in pain and that it is not simply a question of a present-moment need, but they do not know what to do. The nature of body memory is that it is not static, but may be more or less dormant or active depending on external stimuli. A common example of this is when clothing is pulled over a baby's head, activating the memory of passing through the cervix. When babies are tired, body memories are also more likely to be activated. This may resonate with the theme of exhaustion in Stage 3 of the birth process, or it may simply be that the baby becomes more aware of their internal body state and less distracted by interesting objects in the environment. We probably all have had the experience of beginning to drift into sleep at the end of the day and, as we do so, beginning to notice aches or pains that we had not been aware of in the day. Or suddenly jerking awake as some anxiety left over from the day reasserts itself. Babies are no different and may suddenly startle awake just as they are beginning to drift off.

Babies and pain

As well as the emotional content of body memories and their activation, compressed cranial bones and tense connective tissue may be the source of present-moment physical pain. Until recently it was believed that babies did not experience pain as adults do. This led to babies being operated on without the use of anaesthesia as recently as the 1980s (Chamberlain 1998, pp.200–201). Even now, babies are subject to many invasive and painful interventions during and after birth as if they were insensible to the pain. However, a recent study from Oxford University shows that newborns are actually more sensitive to pain than adults (Goksan *et al.* 2015). Using functional magnetic resonance imaging (fMRI) to monitor the brains of babies and adults, they observed the centres of the brain associated with pain that were activated by poking the feet with a pencil. The babies' pain centres responded to pokes that were four times weaker than those that stimulated the same response in adults. This supports what is clearly observable in clinical practice, which is that babies experience pain at birth and also afterwards as the result of painful and stressful medical interventions.

Emotional and physical pain are tolerable for only so long. If there is no relief from suffering it can lead to resignation and dissociation. If babies are met with inappropriate responses to their crying, such as when memory crying is continually responded to as if it were a hunger cry, or they are left to cry on their own, then not only is the original trauma unacknowledged, but it is also overlaid with the frustration of not being understood. The use of controlled crying, in which babies are left for short periods to cry on their own, with ongoing gradual incremental extensions, is promoted by some 'experts' as helping babies to find 'contentment' (Ford 2006). Whilst there may be some short-term benefits from this practice, as parents get a break from the cycles of distress they have been trying unsuccessfully to manage, babies' experience is more often that of being abandoned in their pain. Babies become quiet not because they are now content, but because they have dissociated from their unbearable experience. This is known as 'Good Baby Syndrome' (Appleton 2013a) and shows up in regressive sessions with adults as a source of poor self-esteem, existential anxiety, low energy states such as chronic fatigue, and the underlying belief 'I can never get my needs met', which may get acted out in unhealthy relationship dynamics.

Integrative Baby Therapy

Parents bring their babies for treatment for a number of different reasons. These include inconsolable crying, so-called 'colic', sleep problems, fractious behaviour, or simply because they would like to know if their baby has been left with any after-effects from the birth. For most parents the understanding that babies have experience in the womb or at birth which may impact on them and be the source of their distress is new. As such it needs to be addressed sensitively, without putting pressure on the parents' belief systems or evoking parental guilt (such as 'I hurt my baby' or 'I was not able to protect my baby'). The initial focus therefore is not specifically on the baby, but to build trust and foster a therapeutic alliance with the parents. This involves making them comfortable, both physically and emotionally, getting clear about what they would like from the session and what the therapy can offer. There is no particular sequence in which this unfolds. Rather, the therapist needs to sense what needs attention so as to create ease and openness between the parents and the therapist.

After these preliminaries the therapeutic intention is to open up 'potential space'. This term was originally used by the child analyst D.W. Winnicott (Winnicott 1971, p.107) to describe the space between the mother and baby whereby the baby's sense of self develops out of the reciprocity of the relationship. Here it is used to indicate the space in which the parents and the baby are able to bring their experience. The parents are invited to tell in their own words the stories about what the birth and pregnancy were like for them. For many parents, even though they may have talked for many hours prior to the birth about their hopes and intentions, it is often the first time following the birth that they actually get to hear each other's experience. With all the busyness of adapting to the needs of the baby, this often does not get the time that it deserves. Strong emotions may emerge as the stories are told. The parents are supported to allow the feelings to be part of the therapeutic process. Sometimes as stories are recounted the baby will, at a specific point, begin to memory cry. The parents are then supported to listen to the baby's story.

The potential space allows the 'inherent treatment plan' to emerge (Becker 1997). This term was coined by cranial osteopath Rollin Becker to describe the capacity for the body to move towards its own solution to a symptom, which the physician need only support. The same principle is at work in the 'relational field' that is created by the family and the therapist through the process of deep empathic listening. The therapist does not take on the role of the expert who has answers, but, to use another osteopathic term, becomes the 'fulcrum' or the 'still point' around which the inherent treatment plan can unfold. This requires the therapist to be fully present and tracking what is happening in the relational field to see what needs attention from moment to moment. This is done with the awareness that something very 'intelligent' is trying to happen within the relational field, that will only emerge in its own time. The therapist must resist the temptation to intervene too soon. Only then can the 'prominent presenter' emerge. Karlton Terry describes the 'prominent presenter' as 'the affect most convincingly and repeatedly given by the baby's body language, requesting that the therapy be guided and oriented by the most prominent and persistent theme that is expressed by the baby' (Terry 2009, p.19). Here the term is expanded to include the parents. Often babies need a parent to deregulate their own stress level to create the potential space in which the baby feels it is safe enough to deepen into his or her own 'story'. So the unresolved trauma of a parent may become the prominent presenter. It is indicative of the sensitivity of babies to the relational field that they may wait until a parent has worked through a traumatic issue before beginning to express BBL.

Babies may also respond to a parent talking about a specific stage in the birth, or prenatal event, by expressing the BBL associated with that stage. The baby is clearly resonating with what the parent is saying and feeling. This is a cue to pay attention to the baby and see what the baby has to show us about the experience. All work in Integrative Baby Therapy is based on permission. So the therapist might ask the parents, 'Would it be OK if we paid attention to your baby now?' This both reassures the parents that nothing will be done to their baby without their permission, whilst also inviting the parents to become curious about what their baby is expressing.

Using touch and palpation

Knowing the terrain of the birth and prenatal stages helps to focus this curiosity. For example, if we can see that the baby is touching a specific conjunct site on the lie-side, we can determine exactly where the baby became stuck in the birth process. But, rather than give a lot of information to the parents, the therapist can use this to evoke the interest of the parent by saying something such as, 'I notice little Johnny keeps touching the same spot on the left side of the cranium. I wonder if he's feeling something there?' By drawing the parents into the process the therapist is inviting a deeper empathy on their part, whilst opening the way to suggest possible ways of deepening the exploration of what is happening. This might involve asking permission to palpate the conjunct site. This is done by moving a hand over the conjunct site just off the body. Babies are incredibly open and sensitive. They often respond to even the subtlest palpation. It may be that each time the therapist's hand passes over the conjunct site the BBL becomes more intense or the baby begins to memory cry. This enables the parents to see that the baby is responding to something that is clearly not a present-moment need. Only later or at the end of the session might it be helpful to share a more detailed description of lie-side theory or of the specific birth/prenatal stage that the BBL was indicating.

Once the prominent presenter has clarified, the parents are encouraged to identify the emotional tone. This evokes a more accurate empathy on their part, which the baby feels. Rather than feeling powerless to help a baby who seems to be crying for no particular reason, parents are now able to identify 'when my baby touches that particular place on the head she cries and looks angry'. The anger is now identified with a specific historic experience, which makes sense to the parents. Parents are then supported to empathically mirror the emotion. This is usually modelled first by the therapist, who speaks directly to the baby: 'I can see you are really angry.' This may be expanded to include a reference to what the BBL is telling us, such as: 'That was really painful when you got stuck there' or 'That really frightened you when the medication came through your umbilical cord.'

Allowing babies to tell their stories

Often the crying will initially intensify when we mirror the baby's experience. We have probably all had the experience of telling a friend of something that has been bothering us, and in the telling, *if the listener is really present without trying to find solutions*, we deepen into the story, feeling it more as we tell it. When we have finished there is a sense of relief. It is the same for babies. Supporting parents to be able to tolerate the crying in the session becomes the therapist's primary task at this stage. If the parents' tolerance threshold is dropping, the therapist may look at ways to support them, including various breathing or body awareness techniques, offering support through physical contact, verbal assurances or taking a break from the process. Staying in empathic resonance with the baby as the crying intensifies is usually the most challenging part of the session for the parents. This is partly because the parent naturally wants to soothe the baby and partly because the parents' own unresolved pre- and perinatal trauma may be stimulated. Once the baby has passed through the apex of the crying, it begins to quieten and the baby settles. Parents usually report that their babies cry much less after a session and that it is then more often related to present-moment needs, rather than a body memory. The BBL associated with the memory is also reduced in its intensity or disappears completely. Insofar as memory crying and BBL continues, parents are able to respond with the appropriate empathy so that the baby is more able to move through the experience and settle again. This increases parental confidence and enables a deeper bonding to happen than when both parents and baby are permanently stressed and exhausted.

Empathic mirroring and the capacity to hear the baby's 'story' is at the core of Integrative Baby Therapy. Other therapeutic interventions may also be employed to support babies to complete processes that they were not able to do at the time. This might have been due to overwhelming pain and distress, which caused them to dissociate, or the effects of medication given in the birth, such as induction, augmentation or pain-relieving drugs. Babies will often spontaneously re-enact their birth during a session, moving into the position where they became stuck or overwhelmed. Supporting them to find their own internal impulse to move through this stage, but this time with the conscious support and empathy of the therapist and parents, enables the baby to move through this 'scary place' in an empowered way. As such, it changes the experience. What was initially experienced as overwhelming and fearful is now experienced as a challenge that can be overcome. Supporting the baby's feet to help them build the internal impulse to push forward, whilst empathically tracking and reflecting back their experience, is one such way of doing this. There are numerous other empowering interventions that may be offered in response to the specific BBL and emotional tone that is being expressed.

CASE STUDY

N was six months old when his parents brought him for treatment. They were concerned that he did not seem comfortable in his body, as if he was 'straining against something'. He also went through bouts of high-pitched crying that would only cease when he had exhausted himself. Both parents were present in the sessions. They were both aware that N was trying to communicate something that they were 'not getting'. The father was a little dissociated during the sessions, whilst the mother was very stressed with a strong tendency to self-criticism, which extended to her mothering skills. Both were very eager to do their best to understand and support N, and both parents also had individual therapy sessions at different stages over the next couple of years to work with these issues.

They had both very much wanted a baby and were overjoyed to discover they had conceived after years of trying. They had hoped for a water birth at home, but as N was late in terms of the due date, they were persuaded to go into hospital where induction drugs were given. Pethidine was given to relieve the labour pains. After this the birth proceeded very quickly, but with N becoming stuck whilst crowning. His mother felt shocked by the speed and intensity of the birth. It seemed to her that N was still very 'doped up' by the pethidine after the birth and that the hospital staff tried to force him to latch on when neither of them were ready to breast-feed. After this there were a number of feeding problems and he needed to be fed initially with a syringe. However, they were later able to establish breastfeeding.

During the first session N took my hand a number of times, pressed my fingers hard into his umbilical area and then pushed my hand away. Each time he did this he held his breath, arching his back and straining, as if he was trying to push something out through his abdomen. As the parents were very open to the possibility that N was showing us something that he had experienced during the birth, I felt able to relate to them that what I was seeing was that he was telling us something about how he had experienced what had come through the umbilical cord.

As he also began to rotate to his right, which was his lie-side, it suggested that this was associated with his birth experience. The particular intensity and rhythm of his expressions were also congruent with the nature of induction drugs, which instigate much stronger and longer contractions than natural physiological contractions. This particular intensity and rhythm can be seen in many babies whose births have been induced or augmented. As he moved into the rotational phase of birth N expressed anger, both with his eyes and in his crying. There was also a quality of ambivalence about moving forward, as if he was being pushed before he was ready. Many children and adults whose births were augmented or induced are very sensitive to having their own pacing over-ridden later in life, and may experience even the most gentle encouragement as a forceful manipulation (Emerson 1996, p.76).

In this session both the parents and myself were able to empathize with N's anger. Also, in being able to pull my finger into and away from his umbilicus, N was able to regulate his experience of what was coming into this area in a way he had not been able to do during the birth. At the end of the session his body was more relaxed and he was happy to breast-feed. When they arrived for the following session a week later the parents reported that N had 'matured enormously', was 'more vocal' and that his head and face had 'changed shape'. The high-pitched crying had disappeared, as had the sense of straining.

N presented in the second session as being more relaxed, with less compression held in his cranium along the lie-side. In this session he moved spontaneously into the rotation stage (Stage 2) of his birth, where he became very disoriented and anxious. This seemed more connected with the effects of the pethidine as he moved through the mid-pelvis. The effects of pethidine are that babies feel disconnected from their mothers, leaving them feeling alone, whilst at the same time their own awareness becomes clouded and diminished by the effects of the drug (Emerson 1996, p.48). In therapy sessions, as one layer of pre- and perinatal experience is worked through, another will often present itself to be worked through. This is always led by the inherent treatment plan which unfolds as the baby prioritizes what needs to be worked with. *It is never dictated by the therapist.* Having resolved the layer of experience connected with the induction drugs, N now needed to work with the effects of the pethidine and the disorientation of Stage 2.

After this session, in which N was supported to feel reconnected with his mother, the parents reported 'huge developmental developments' and the subjective sense that N was 'more embodied'.

We worked together for another nine sessions, at first on a weekly basis, then fortnightly, then monthly. During this time N continued to show BBL and memory crying, sometimes moving rapidly between a birth stage and a prenatal phase, when there was an experiential theme linking the two. The predominant prenatal theme that he worked with was implantation. This is when the blastocyst implants into the uterus wall and has its first taste of the maternal blood. He showed this through a very specific body gesture that is associated with this phase. This involves a burrowing motion with the forehead, either into a pillow or the mother's body, along with a pulsatory movement that is expressed throughout the whole body. He also threw himself violently at his mother, smashing into her with a particular force and angrily biting her. When these sorts of aggressive expressions accompany the implantation BBL they tend to reflect the blastocyst's experience of meeting the uterine tissues. It can seem bizarre at first that such early cellular experiences have an impact that is then carried into later life, but clinical experience confirms this. In this case, even though N's parents very much wanted a baby, his mother held a lot of historical stress which was exacerbated by the need to be the 'perfect mother'. This was held in her tissues and it seemed that N was telling us something about his encounter with this quality in her.

In the present moment there was also a rather harsh way in which she handled him, that lacked softness. Over a number of sessions we worked with this by encouraging her to protect herself, whilst still allowing N to express his feelings, and to handle him more gently. She was also able to express to him her feelings of regret that she had not been able to receive him more gently when he first arrived in the womb. These feelings very much arose as an intuitive response to his actions, as opposed to any interpretation by the therapist. The combination of empathy for N, self-care by the mother and change in quality of contact resulted in less aggressive behaviour in N, and a ceasing of the implantation BBL. However, as she tended to be very self-critical and masochistic in regard to how she dealt with these issues, it was suggested that she have some extra support for herself. It was at this stage that she began a series of craniosacral therapy and psychotherapy sessions, which helped her to soften these tendencies. This enabled her to be more appropriately available for N.

Writing later of the sessions with N she wrote that they 'presented a remarkable opportunity to deepen our understanding and compassion both within and outside of the family. The sessions allowed N to express at a fundamental and pre-verbal level how he experienced his entry into the world and with guidance we have learnt how to recognize and respond to his "voice". He has grown into a child who can and does communicate very clearly, often showing levels of understanding about relationship that is surprising. His communication is accompanied with a confidence of "being" in the world, and feeling free. It is very clear to us that this stems from the space created by these sessions in which he experienced the world as a place that supports, listens and acknowledges' (Appleton 2013b).

Conclusion

In conclusion, babies reveal their prenatal and birth experience through BBL and memory crying. These 'stories' mostly go unheard. Clinical experience shows that being able to 'hear' and respond to these stories empathically brings relief to symptoms such as inconsolable crying, fractiousness and sleep disturbances. As well as symptomatic relief it supports deeper contact and bonding between babies and their parents. As indicated in the words of N's mother above, it may also engender greater communication skills, self-confidence and empathy.

References

Agustoni, A. (2013) *Craniosacral Therapy for Children*. Berkeley, CA: North Atlantic Books.

Appleton, M. (2013a) 'Good Baby Syndrome.' *Juno. A Natural Approach to Family Life*. Issue 32. Bristol: Juno Publishing.

Appleton, M. (2013b) 'Craniosacral Therapy for Babies, Children and Families.' *Juno. A Natural Approach to Family Life*. Issue 34. Bristol: Juno Publishing.

Barrett, S. (2013) *Secrets of Your Cells*. Boulder, CO: Sounds True.

Becker, R.E. (1997) *Life in Motion*. Portland, OR: Rudra Press.

Chamberlain, D. (1998) *The Mind of Your Newborn Baby*. Berkeley, CA: North Atlantic Books.

Chamberlain, D. (2013) *Windows to the Womb. Revealing the Conscious Baby from Conception to Birth*. Berkeley, CA: North Atlantic Books.

Emerson, W. (1996) *Birth Trauma. The Psychological Effects of Obstetrical Interventions*. Petaluma, CA: Emerson Training Seminars.

Emerson, W. (2000) *Collected Works 2. The Pre- and Perinatal Treatment of Children and Adults*. Petaluma, CA: Emerson Training Seminars.

Emerson, W. (2004a) *The Emerson Perinatal Stages Manual*. Petaluma, CA: Emerson Training Seminars.

Emerson, W. (2004b) *The Emerson Prenatal Stages Manual*. Petaluma, CA: Emerson Training Seminars.

Fodor, N. (1949) *The Search for the Beloved*. New York: Hermitage Press.

Ford, G. (2006) *The Complete Sleep Guide for Contented Babies and Toddlers*. London: Vermilion.

Gabriel, M., and Gabriel, M. (1995) *Remembering Your Life Before Birth*. Santa Rosa, CA: Aslan.

Goksan, S., Hartley, C., Emery, F., Cockrill, N., *et al.* (2015) 'fMRI reveals neural activity overlap between adult and infant pain.' *Elife 4*. doi:10.7554/elife.06356.

Grof, S. (1976) *Realms of the Human Unconscious. Observations from LSD Research*. New York: Dutton.

Grof, S., and Grof, C. (2010) *Holotropic Breathwork*. New York: State University of New York Press.

Ho, M.-W. (1998) *The Rainbow and the Worm. The Physics of Organisms*. New Jersey, London, Singapore and Hong Kong: World Scientific.

Laing, R.D. (1976) *The Facts of Life*. Harmondsworth: Penguin Books.

Lake, F. (1966) *Clinical Theology*. London: Darton, Longman & Todd.

Larimore, T. and Farrant, G. (1995) 'Universal body movements in cellular consciousness and what they mean.' *Primal Renaissance 1*, 1. International Primal Association.

Oschman, J. (2000) *Energy Medicine. The Scientific Basis* (8th edition). Edinburgh and New York: Churchill Livingstone.

Pearshall, P. (1988) *The Heart's Code*. Wellingborough: Thorsons.

Peirsman, E., and Peirsman, N. (2006) *Craniosacral Therapy for Babies and Small Children*. Berkeley, CA: North Atlantic Books.

Rank, O. (1929) *The Trauma of Birth*. New York: Harcourt Brace.

Share, L. (1994) *If Someone Speaks, It Gets Lighter. Dreams and the Reconstruction of Infant Trauma.* Hillsdale, NJ: Analytic Press.

Terry, K. (2005) *The Sperm Journey/The Egg Journey.* Institute of Pre- and Perinatal Education.

Terry, K. (2009) *Baby Therapy Course. Class 1 Notes.* Institute of Pre- and Perinatal Education.

Upledger, J. (1990) *SomatoEmotional Release and Beyond.* Palm Beach, FL: UI Publishing.

Upledger, J. (1996) *A Brain Is Born: Exploring the Birth and Development of the Central Nervous System.* Berkeley, CA: North Atlantic Books.

Verny, T. (2014) 'What cells remember: Toward a unified field theory of memory.' *Journal of Prenatal and Perinatal Psychology and Health 29,* 1, 13–16.

Winnicott, D.W. (1971) *Playing and Reality.* London and New York: Tavistock/Routledge.

CHAPTER 6

PRENATAL UMBILICAL AFFECT
THE GREAT PRENATAL CONUNDRUM

Matthew Appleton

The prenatal environment

Psychodynamic theories of personality development generally assume that the period prior to birth is of little or no significance. The result of this omission is that in the therapy room a vast territory of human experience is not acknowledged or welcomed in the therapeutic relationship and, as such, is not brought into consciousness. The same is true for babies in their relationship with parents and medical professionals. This means that they have to bear this experience on their own. It cannot be brought into relationship and so it is not mirrored back in a meaningful way. If we talk about a difficult childhood experience that is empathically mirrored back to us, we feel acknowledged both in the impact of the experience and our capacity to survive it. For example, if as a child I was beaten, and later in life I am able to talk about this in therapy, there is some relief of the emotional tension associated with the original event, and I am also able to explore subsequent behaviours that have arisen out of this experience. This might include an appreciation of my resilience in the face of such adversity, as well as an understanding of anxiety-based behaviours that limit my capacity to be in present-day relationships.

If I had to bear this experience on my own, without the opportunity to bring it into consciousness, I would only know it as an unfathomable tension and inner pain, with associated patterns of behaviour that appeared irrational, infantile or destructive. This in turn would undermine my self-esteem, especially as these behaviours would also be reflected back to me as 'bad', 'stupid' or 'crazy' by teachers, as I grew up, or, later in life, by colleagues, friends and lovers. I would not feel understood or understand myself. This is the experience of most people in relation to their prenatal experience. It remains both in the personal and cultural shadow as unconscious experience that informs all subsequent experience. This is especially true of the umbilical relationship between the prenate[1] and the mother. It is the template for all other relationships: parental, social, intimate and environmental. Our embodied 'feeling tone' of who we are and what the world is like arises out of this most formative of relationships. Our essential beliefs about our self-worth and how safe we are in the world emerge out of this internal sensory milieu.

The great prenatal conundrum

The term 'umbilical affect' is used to describe the 'feeling state of the foetus as brought about by blood reaching him through the umbilical vein' (Moss 1987, p.203). Prenatal umbilical affect includes the experience of external toxins mediated through the maternal blood and the feeling tones of the mother. Toxins may include environmental pollution (car fumes, industrial waste), medication and recreational drugs (including cigarettes, caffeine and alcohol), food preservatives, heavy metals, leakage from tooth fillings, paint fumes, deodorants and hairsprays, poor nutrition, and so on. One recent US study detected 287 commercial chemicals, pesticides and pollutants in the umbilical cord blood taken from ten randomly selected newborn infants (Houlihan *et al.* 2005, p.5).

The maternal 'feeling tones' include the mother's feelings about being pregnant, her relationships with her wider social circle and support network (partner, other children, family, community, country), her financial concerns, her own self-image, illness and any distressing or shocking events she may encounter. These may include moving home, the loss or serious illness of a friend or family member, violence or witnessing a violent event either personally or via the media, such as a terrorist atrocity. These will be transmitted to the foetus via shifts in hormonal and neuropeptide activity. The mother's psychological and emotional history is also an underlying factor.

---

1   The term 'prenate' is used here as a generic term for both the embryonic and foetal stages of prenatal life.

This is embodied in her capacity to adapt to stressful situations and the baseline of stress that she brings to everyday life.

Many studies have shown that prenates respond to maternal stress with their own stress responses. A study of 28 pregnant women in Southern Italy following an earthquake that shook the area discovered that the prenates were in a hyperactive state for between two and eight hours (Chamberlain 2013, p.44). A similar study was conducted of 38 women who were pregnant in September 2001 and who were at or near the World Trade Center at the time of the terrorist attack. Saliva studies showed that those women who went on to develop post-traumatic stress disorder (PTSD) had lower cortisol levels than those who were also exposed but did not develop PTSD. About a year later, the researchers measured cortisol levels in the children, and found that those born to the women who had developed PTSD also had lower levels of the hormone compared with the children whose mothers did not develop PTSD (*Guardian* 2011). A study in San Francisco revealed that the babies of mothers who were unhappy about their pregnancy, or the prospect of motherhood, showed increased signs of 'upset' as compared with those who were born to mothers who were happy to be pregnant (Montagu 1965, p.153). These are just a few random studies from a much larger body of research.

Umbilical affect can range from 'positive' to 'strongly negative' as maternal moods and environmental stresses come and go (Maret 1997, pp.25–26). Prenates are resilient and able to adapt to short-term negative umbilical affect. Encountering some negative affect may even be 'educational' for the prenate (Maret 1997, p.28). Knowing that s/he may encounter difficulty, that it can be managed and will pass, helps prepare the prenate for birth and the demands of the external environment. It helps build resilience through a toning of prenatal defensive systems. However, chronic or severe negative umbilical affect can overwhelm the prenate's capacity to integrate the experience. This is often experienced as being flooded by a sense of 'toxicity' or 'badness'. The 'great prenatal conundrum' is how to minimize the impact of chronic or severe negative umbilical affect whilst still keeping the life-line of the umbilical cord open enough to survive. Whereas prenates thrive with the influx of positive umbilical affect, with chronic or severe negative umbilical affect survival becomes the priority. Prenates are extremely resourceful in the survival strategies they adopt to manage negative umbilical affect. In the short term these bring relief. However, the long-term consequence of needing to defend against what is experienced as a stressful or toxic environment is that the adaption becomes a way of life. Prenatal survival strategies form the basis for dealing with later stresses and relational difficulties. They can also inhibit the capacity to be open and receptive to the 'goodness of life'.

Inner motility[2] as an expression of health

Amoeba are single-celled organisms which consist of a membrane, protoplasm and a nucleus. Studies of amoeba under the microscope reveal that they expand out to their environment when it is nurturing for them, for example if there is food. If something toxic enters into their environment they contract away from it. If they are not able to escape this toxicity the contraction remains, building up a great deal of inner tension. If there is no possibility of relief from this, the membrane thickens, as if to create a stronger barrier against the world, and the protoplasm becomes cloudy as its lack of motility reduces its capacity to metabolize waste products and take in fresh nutrition. If the contraction is chronic and severe enough, the membrane and nucleus begin to break apart. The amoeba can no longer hold its integrity (Baker 1967, pp.3–6).

Although as human beings we are more complex than the amoeba, our essential physiological make-up is of a membrane (the skin), protoplasm (cellular cytoplasm and extra-cellular fluid) and a nucleus (the autonomic nervous system). Like the amoeba we may also be conditioned through our prenatal experience to either contract away from the world which is experienced as unpleasant, or expand out to it with the expectation of being welcomed and needs being met. The essential condition of chronic contraction is experienced as an underlying sense of anxiety, whereas the capacity to expand out to the world is experienced as pleasure and expresses itself as an ability to fully embrace life. Mediated in human beings through the autonomic nervous system, the tendency for chronic contraction forms the predisposition for many health problems later in life (Odent 1986). Accompanied by bouts of over-expansion, perhaps mediated through alcohol, drugs or outbursts of aggression or hysteria, many behavioural and social problems have their roots in these attempts to be free of this underlying inner tension (Reich 1942).

---

2   The term 'motility' is used in biology to refer to an organism's ability to express movement freely.

Babies who become stuck in contracted states may be experienced as fractious or diagnosed with 'colic'. During Integrative Baby Therapy (IBT) sessions 'fractious' or 'colicky' babies often take the therapist's hand and pull the fingers into the umbilicus, whilst at the same time emitting a cough, cry or guttural sound that conveys a sense of inner tension. This is Baby Body Language (BBL) (see Chapter 5) which indicates that an unresolved umbilical issue is active in maintaining the contraction. Insofar as this is empathically mirrored, the baby is able to discharge tension and relax. When it is not empathically mirrored the tension remains and becomes chronically anchored in the connective tissues of the body. Tight connective tissues, along with autonomic imbalances, maintain levels of inner pressure, contributing to conditions such as hypertension, breathing and digestive problems, poor posture, headaches and migraines, chronic fatigue, impaired impulse control and emotional difficulties (Upledger 1990). Therapeutic work with adults where BBL associated with umbilical themes is present supports the proposition that chronic or severe negative umbilical affect can be a predisposing factor in many health issues.

For example, a male client exploring the sensations related to a conflict with his wife became aware of a strong contraction around his umbilicus. As he deepened into his embodied experience he became aware of an underlying panic, which gave rise to a pulling up of his knees in a self-protective gesture. As he became familiar with these sensations over a number of sessions, he was able to link them with a long-term digestive disorder, chronic lower back tension and tense legs, which, in turn, made him susceptible to knee and ankle injuries. He also had a deep fear of 'getting it wrong' for women, with an underlying rage towards his wife, which erupted as a defence against his vulnerability. In regressive therapy sessions he was able to trace this back to his experience in the womb and his mother's desire to abort him. Although it would be presumptuous to say that the prenatal experience was the *cause* of his present-day problems, it would be equally presumptuous to dismiss his formative womb experience as anything less than a powerful contributing factor.

If we consider that early interventions with babies might alleviate the development of subsequent physical and emotional problems later in life, then we can view such interventions as preventative, as well as relieving stress for parents and babies in the present moment. Such correlations would be hard to quantify, as we can only assume predispositions towards health or disease.

Later life events will either consolidate these so as to create specific symptoms or will alleviate those tendencies. Nevertheless, work with adults in regressive therapy reveals that many health conditions are derived from, and maintained by, specific patterns of tension related to prenatal umbilical stress and birth-related issues. Early interventions with babies reduce or dissolve these tension patterns, allowing the possibility of greater inner motility and freedom as a baseline for future growth and experience (Appleton 2014, pp.41–55).

Prenatal womb experience

It is generally assumed that prenates are insensible in the womb or suspended in a somnolent state in which consciousness gradually emerges. However, in recent decades more and more evidence from improved scanning technologies has revealed how active and responsive to their environment prenates are (Chamberlain 2013). In IBT sessions babies reveal through their BBL how active they were in utero at mediating negative umbilical affect. If prenatal life was very stressful, babies may behave as if they were still in the womb, defending themselves as best they can against the onslaught of negative umbilical affect. They are stuck in their survival strategies, not knowing that it is safe enough for them to relax. This may be because some of the stresses that were present prenatally are still present. Babies are very open and sensitive to their parents' emotional states and stress levels. In IBT we refer to the 'family field'. This is the immediate environment that is created by the interactions of the individual family members. We all have the experience of walking into a room and immediately sensing a certain atmosphere. It may be one of warmth that we *feel* invites us in, or perhaps one of tension or anger which does not feel comfortable and puts us into a state of alert apprehension. We sense something is wrong. Babies are exquisitely tuned into such atmospheres and the family field functions like an extended womb. This is especially true for most of the first year of life, as the baby is totally dependent on his or her family to regulate his stress levels. The baby responds to this extended womb as if still in the physical womb, and the archaic survival strategies learnt in utero are the learned ways by which the baby continues to defend against what is perceived as a hostile or unsafe environment.

Even if the family field is relatively stress-free, babies may still be stuck in prenatal survival strategies. This can simply be due to the fact that their experience has not been empathically mirrored in a way that allows them to release the inner tension. An adult version of this might be arriving at a friend's house after a stressful or frightening encounter, such as being threatened by a stranger, or knocked off a bike. We would need to tell our story of the experience before we could begin to relax. As we did so our emotions would come to the surface – we might cry and shake. In doing so the inner tension associated with the experience would diminish. The capacity of the friend to understand, empathize and be present with our distress would determine how much stress we could release. If the friend, instead of listening, seemed preoccupied with their own concerns, distracted by something else, or began offering possible solutions without really listening, we would not feel that we have been heard and the tension would remain. If the friend, instead of listening, tried to distract us by offering us inappropriate diversions, such as something to eat, not only would we feel unheard, but we would very likely either become enraged with the friend or begin to doubt our own sanity. When parents, even with the best intentions, respond to memory crying (see Chapter 5) as if it were a present-moment need such as hunger or tiredness, babies respond the same way as we might as adults. Initially they become very angry, but in time may give up on getting the environmental response they need (Appleton 2013).

Prenatal survival strategies

There are a number of strategies prenates use to mediate negative umbilical affect. These are more or less effective depending on the degree and duration of the stress and the stage in the pregnancy that it is experienced. First trimester babies have fewer options than second or third trimester babies and are also more vulnerable because their organs are still forming. As the various organs form at different times, the forming organs/structures are more likely to be impacted by negative umbilical affect that occurs during that time. This is because the prenate's blood supply prioritizes the emerging organ to supply it with the nutrition it needs to develop (Terry 2011, p.17).

The various survival strategies that babies call upon in utero live on in their BBL. These can be clearly observed as records of prenatal life that continue to exist post-birth. The following examples are the most common forms of BBL related to prenatal umbilical themes.

Pinching

The abdominal muscles are contracted to squeeze the umbilical cord as it enters the abdomen. This works with the natural flexion of the prenate and is especially utilized in the first trimester, when there are fewer options. As with any of these strategies, pinching can only slow down the influx of negative umbilical affect. It cannot stop it completely, as to completely cut off the maternal blood supply would be suicide. However, it does enable the prenate to some degree to regulate the amount of 'badness' that is flooding his or her body at times of heightened stress.

Arching

The prenate arches (Figure 6.1) against the influx of 'badness'. This is more effective in the third trimester, when the prenate is able to push with the legs to support the pushing out through the umbilicus from the mid-lumbar region of the back. This arching is often seen in babies diagnosed with colic. The muscles of the lumbar region of the back are rigid and the belly is thrust forward, as if trying to push something away. Digestive difficulties are most often mistaken as the cause of this discomfort and distress, instead of being one of the symptoms of the inner tension that the body is still holding onto. Supporting the feet to give power to the impulse to push away that comes through the legs, along with empathic mirroring, generally results in a release of tension and a resolution of the digestive problems.

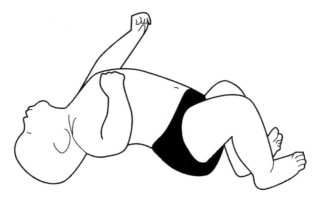

Figure 6.1 Baby arching

There are several forms of arching recognised in Integrative Baby Therapy. In relation to umbilical affect the arching involves what appears to be an active pushing out from the navel, as if trying to push something away.

Pedalling and conducting

This can be seen in babies as frantic movements of the limbs as if s/he is conducting an orchestra with the arms and pedalling a bike with the legs (Figure 6.2). These movements speed up the circulation of negative umbilical affect through the body and its exit through the umbilical arteries, which arise from the groin and spiral out around the central umbilical vein. This strategy may be present in the first trimester, as well as later in gestation, as the limb buds may be actively used in this strategy.

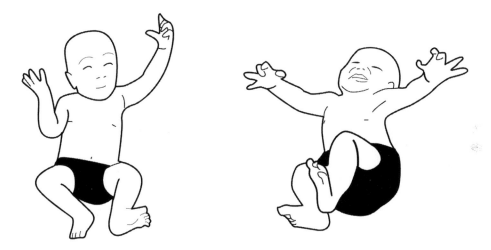

Figure 6.2 Baby pedalling and conducting

Cord squeezing

Once the hands are fully formed and able to grasp (in the third to fourth month), they can be utilized to squeeze the cord, thus regulating the amount of flow that comes through it.

Umbilical shunting

Either as a function of the protoplasm in early embryological development or later using the diaphragm, the prenate 'shunts' 'badness' or 'toxicity' into the lower body. This is to prioritize protection of the major organs of the upper body (head and heart). If the diaphragm, as a protective boundary, is overridden, the prenate will contract around the throat, then the jaw and cranial base in an attempt to protect the brain.

Hemispheric shunting

When shunting into the lower body is ineffective, the prenate prioritizes the 'whole' by sacrificing parts. Initially this involves shunting badness and toxicity to one side. The mechanism by which this is done is not understood, but we can assume it is a function of the protoplasm. When this strategy is overwhelmed, the prenate will shunt the negative umbilical affect into specific organs, creating pockets of 'badness'.

Dissociation

When all other strategies are exhausted, the prenate's only option is dissociation. The sensations are so overwhelmingly terrible that the prenate 'freezes' and numbs so as not to feel anything. This can be thought of as a kind of dying, in that the embodied experience of aliveness is diminished. In later life any external stress that stimulates the body memory of the prenatal anguish can provoke the sense 'I would rather die' than feel so terrible.

Metaphoric Umbilical Mouth Movements and breathing patterns

Archaic expressions of the prenate's experience of umbilical affect can also be observed in mouth movements and breathing patterns. Pre- and perinatal educator Karlton Terry refers to these expressive mouth movements as 'Metaphoric Umbilical Mouth Movements' (MUMMs). As the umbilical cord and the mouth have similar functions in that they both are involved with taking in oxygen and nutrition and expelling waste such as carbon dioxide, there is a 'neurological resonance' between them. According to Terry: 'As the neurology of the prenate matures it catches up with the pre-existing biological conditions, and neuronal nets begin firing in the brain' (Terry 2011, p.32). As well as being simply functional, the prenate's relationship with the cord is intimate and expressive. The expressive movements that we associate with the mouth, tongue and throat are already present in the prenate's relationship with the cord. Sucking in, spitting out, slurping, blocking, licking, deflecting and yearning are all there as expressive plasmatic movements of the prenate in relation to the cord. The most prevailing and powerful tones of umbilical affect will lay down the densest neural networks, which generate habitual ways of interfacing with our environment. Once the cord is cut these expressive movements are taken up by the mouth and its associated structures as habitual motion patterns. Breathing styles interact with MUMMs, showing patterns of holding on and letting go that reflect the prenate's experience of letting in and blocking at the umbilicus. These basic primitive survival functions associated with breathing, nutrition and expelling waste are conditioned by our experience in utero and remain as expressive tendencies throughout life.

Some of the common MUMMs and/or breathing patterns include the following.

Licking
This occurs when something nice is experienced in the environment. It is not simply the licking of lips when smelling food or presented with something tasty to eat. The tongue flicks out and may flick to the side, as if something nurturing or pleasant is detected at the periphery. This may also reflect, later in life, an attitude of not being able to get needs met directly, but in a 'sideways' manner. Often when making a suggestion that appeals to a client this little flick of the tongue appears, signifying that it appeals to the client ('It tastes good').

Blocking
The lips are drawn tightly together. The gesture is a defensive one that signifies 'nothing will get past here'. The breath is either held or shallow whilst the blocking is in place (Figure 6.3). It signifies a 'no' to whatever is being experienced in the environment. People who find it hard to express their 'no' verbally may agree to something verbally whilst exhibiting blocking MUMMs. The body speaks the deeper truth.

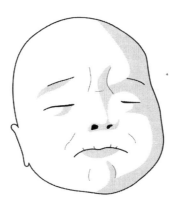

Figure 6.3 Baby blocking

Gulping

The breath may be held for a prolonged period and then a sudden huge gulp is taken. This is expressive of a prenate who had to reduce his or her needs by restricting the influx of maternal blood until there was a reduction of negative umbilical affect and an opportunity for stress-free nutrition arrived. This might occur at a moment when a mother who is generally stressed relaxes. The prenate is not able to trust that this state will continue, so takes in as much 'goodness' as s/he can whilst it is available. This style of managing umbilical affect is later expressed in a tendency to periodically over-indulge, as there is the unconscious belief that it may be the only opportunity. The environment is not trusted as a sustainable resource from which we can take what we need when we need it. All of these conditioned umbilical rhythms and survival strategies are reflected in later life in how we relate to food, money and intimate relationship. Our relationship with the planet as a resource is also an expression of this primal experience. With the gulping strategy there is often the tendency to hoard, which is expressed in the breathing pattern as a holding between gulps.

Straw breathing

The lips are pursed and the breath is drawn in as if through a straw (Figure 6.4). The quality of this breathing style is of having to work hard at drawing in what nutrition is possible. Later in life this appears as a tendency to have to work hard for little reward. An accompanying unconscious belief that is usually associated with this breathing style is that 'I have to reduce my needs to survive'. As an umbilical expression it is rooted in the experience of the prenate whose mother's resources were depleted in some way. This might be emotionally or physically if the mother was ill, for example. It may also be that her diet or environment did not nourish and support her as she needed during the pregnancy. Frank Lake, a pioneer in the field of pre- and perinatal psychology, describes the phenomenon of the 'foetal therapist', whereby the prenate 'feels the need to give to this poor, weak mother. Well aware that it has little to give because little has been received, none the less there can be a fateful sense that "it is my role to keep her alive"' (Lake 1978, p.20). Many people attracted to caring professions or caring roles in the family have a tendency to look after others at the expense of their own needs, often working hard for little reward. Underlying this tendency is the unconscious belief that 'I will not survive if I do not look after others'.

As with all unconscious prenatal survival strategies, behaviour is driven by the early conditioning, and the awareness of other choices is diminished.

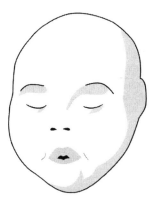

Figure 6.4 Baby straw breathing

Pushing out
Air is expelled from the mouth with force. The lips are usually pursed and the gesture is similar to whistling. There may even be a slight whistle that accompanies the out-breath. This pushing out often appears at a slightly exaggerated pace compared with relaxed breathing, or it may appear after a prolonged period of holding the breath. The in-breath is shallow and may appear almost non-existent. This reproduces the prenate's experience of having to push out as soon as s/he has taken in. It allows a degree of umbilical nutrition to be taken in, whilst defending against taking in too much negative umbilical affect. Along with straw breathing it requires a lot of work for little reward, and both these breathing styles may be present in adults with chronic fatigue.

Coughing
Although coughing is not specifically either a breathing style or a MUMM, it is appropriate to include it here as umbilically related BBL. There is a particular cough that is associated with negative umbilical affect. It is a 'ka-ka' sound and it often starts or becomes more pronounced when the umbilical region is being palpated. It is the body's attempt to clear the imprint of the toxicity or 'badness' that came through the cord. With adults this may be accompanied by the urge to retch. Handing tissues to them, they are encouraged to cough and spit into the tissue, whilst visualizing clearing the negative umbilical affect. They are further encouraged to throw away the

tissue, with the sense of not wanting to carry this imprint within them any more. Images of sticky blackness, sometimes accompanied by an unfamiliar taste, frequently arise in these experiences.

The importance of working with babies

BBL associated with prenatal umbilical survival strategies is extremely common. This reflects a lack of awareness of the importance of the prenatal period in human development and a lack of protection for pregnant women, so as to enable them to experience a peaceful pregnancy. Indigenous cultures that utilize ritual and community support for mother and prenate during pregnancy and birth are marked by their qualities of non-violence and relational acuity (Grille 2005; Maiden and Farwell 1997; Somé 2009). The idea that babies may benefit from therapy is not generally recognized in modern post-industrial cultures, yet clinical experience shows that it can ameliorate many of the difficult conditions that prenates encounter during the gestation period. It also serves to demonstrate the sensitivity and awareness of prenates and newborns, as is communicated through the interaction with babies as they 'tell their stories'. Perhaps, in time, this can serve to awaken an awareness in our society, with its endemic violence and relational dysfunction, the same wisdom demonstrated by those indigenous cultures that recognize the importance of the prenatal period for both individual well-being and community cohesion.

Witnessing the distress of babies who are cycling in their prenatal survival strategies, it is not surprising to the attuned observer that, unchecked, this distress would find expression later in life in disruptive behaviours. The baby is not a poorly developed adult, but a whole person, and the totality of their being is engaged in this struggle. It is by engaging with the baby as a whole person, who already has a lifetime's experience, that the therapist begins to develop a relationship with the baby. The quality of contact that the therapist brings to the session is one of equality and cooperation, not condescending platitudes. This engages the baby's inherent embodied wisdom. It has already been described in Chapter 5 how the session includes and works with the parents, as well as the baby. These principles are at work in any session, whether the prominent theme is prenatal or birth-related.

CASE STUDY

H was six weeks old when his mother brought him for his first session. This was followed by two further sessions. He was three months old at the time of his last session. The father declined to attend the sessions, as he regarded baby care in general as a woman's domain, which had little to do with him. The main reasons for bringing H to therapy were 'colic' and that he pulled away from his mother when she attempted breastfeeding. He had been seen once by a chiropractor, who had identified neck tension and pressure in the cranium. The birth had not been an easy one. The mother had hoped for a water birth at home, but when the waters broke there were no contractions and H's heart rate became accelerated. They were taken to hospital and the birth was induced. During 24 hours of intense contractions the mother was given pethidine, gas and air, and an epidural. When he finally emerged, H had the cord around his neck and the amniotic fluid contained meconium.

The pregnancy had also been stressful. H was the first baby, and the parents had many anxieties about how they would cope. The relationship between them was fraught, with lots of arguments. During the first trimester they moved home, which was very disruptive and stressful. There were also some tensions connected with the mother's own parents, who were very critical of her and her life choices. Her general demeanour was one of holding back her feelings. Although she was clearly tense and at times found the sessions challenging, she found it hard to recognize or articulate her emotions. This meant that a lot of the work in the sessions was oriented towards supporting her to develop inner resources and increase her capacity to tolerate H's emotional expressions. These were predominantly anxiety and sadness. He did not show much anger and had something of the foetal therapist about him. He frequently looked to his mother, not with any sense of reaching out for support, but as if to check that she was still okay. The mother exuded a quality of inner tension that was not simply to do with what H was exhibiting, but had a deeply entrenched quality that had been learnt in childhood. Her own BBL gave clues to the unresolved early trauma that she carried within her.

Although we did some work relating to the cord around the neck and the place where H became stuck in the birth, the most prominent BBL was related to the umbilicus. This included pedalling and conducting, diaphragmatic shunting, umbilical ('ka-ka') coughing, arching, and strongly blocking (tight-lipped) MUMMs. He was very pale and initially avoided eye contact with either myself or his mother. His diaphragm was tight, his pelvis rigid and his chest held in chronic inspiration. He seemed lost in his own world. When his mother did try to embrace him or feed him he stiffened and pulled away. The rejection of contact and the breast can often be traced back to the umbilical relationship and echoes the earlier needing to defend against the mother. At no point did he seem comfortable in his body and his distress was clear. The overall impression I had was of someone who was very alone, who did not expect relief or actively seek it. The mother embodied the same quality, so that the family field felt very disconnected. Building trust and inviting contact were vital prerequisites for working with the umbilical theme.

When there was enough trust and connection to begin work with the BBL, which was mainly in the second session, I began by palpating the umbilical region. Babies are incredibly sensitive to contact in this area, and just bringing the hand close to the area may elicit a response. Even though the physical cord is no longer present, an energetic 'umbilical current' can still be palpated throughout life. It has a pulsatory quality as it spirals out from the umbilicus to the environment and back again. It is clearly palpable, and students who may be initially sceptical are often surprised to feel it and to witness the effects of palpating it. When I palpated H's umbilical current his pedalling and conducting BBL became more frantic. By now he was making clear eye contact with me. There was an imploring quality that invited me to see him and to empathize with his experience. I verbally reflected back to him that I could see his sadness and anxiety. At the same time I encouraged the mother to recognize and name what she saw and felt.

It is not always possible to distinguish what belongs to umbilical affect due to drugs given to the mother at birth and prenatal umbilical affect. However, pedalling and conducting indicate mainly prenatal issues. The quality of isolation also felt as if it belonged to a continuum of which birth had been an intense, but relatively short, episode. However, I emphasized the impact of drugs at birth, as I felt this would be easier for the mother to accept, both because prenatal experience is often harder for parents to comprehend and also because the effect of drugs given at birth is less likely to evoke guilt than the mother's own emotional state as the source of distress. In sessions where this can be named and worked with, a greater accuracy of empathy can be attained and the parents are able to express their regret that their ambivalence or stress was felt by their baby. However, in this instance, I did not feel the mother would be able to tolerate hearing this. For some mothers, even knowing that they were not able to protect their babies at birth from interventions can be a source of guilt. It is a delicate area to explore, and the therapist needs to proceed with caution and sensitivity. At the same time, if the truth cannot be faced, the babies are left holding that experience on their own.

Supporting H's feet as he pedalled empowered his impulse to push away the umbilical affect. All the time I empathically mirrored whatever emotional expression surfaced and also verbally mirrored the coughing. As I did so he looked deeply into my eyes, whereas initially he had avoided any contact. This is another indication that the babies are feeling met in their experience. If we get it wrong they will turn away from eye contact. After just a few minutes his diaphragm began to relax, so that his belly began to breathe for the first time. His pelvis softened and his legs lost their rigidity. His mouth also softened. After one especially strong push through his legs the pedalling and conducting movements stopped. He looked far more relaxed and his eye contact was more inquisitive than avoidant or anxious. Following this session his mother reported that the colic had diminished and he no longer pushed away from her. This made feeding easier and increased her confidence as a mother.

With this easing of symptoms, H's mother decided to stop after the third session. My own impression was that H would benefit from further work, as his BBL was still showing that his umbilical experience was not fully resolved. However, as well as symptom relief, the BBL was less frantic and he was not as lost in the experience as he had been during the first two sessions. This enabled a deeper level of bonding than had previously been possible. Further work may have benefited H with regard to reducing this survival strategy re-emerging during times of stress in the future. Nevertheless, with the work that we did do, if this tendency to contract and withdraw were to emerge again, it would most likely not be as tenacious as if he had not had these sessions.

References

Appleton, M. (2013) 'Good Baby Syndrome.' *Juno. A Natural Approach to Family Life*. Issue 32. Bristol: Juno Publishing.

Appleton, M. (2014) 'Der Einfluss des Geburtstraumas auf das körperliche und seelische Wohlbefinden des Babys.' In S. Hildebrandt, H. Blazy, J. Schacht and W. Bott (eds) *Schwangerschaft und Geburt prägen das Leben*. Heidelberg: Mattes Verlag.

Baker, E.F. (1967) *Man in the Trap*. London and New York: Collier Macmillan.

Chamberlain, D.B. (2013) *Windows to the Womb. Revealing the Conscious Baby from Conception to Birth*. Berkeley, CA: North Atlantic Books.

Grille, R. (2005) *Parenting for a Peaceful World*. Richmond: The Children's Project.

Guardian (2011) *Pregnant 9/11 Survivors Transmitted Trauma to their Children*. Available at www.theguardian.com/science/neurophilosophy/2011/sep/09/pregnant-911-survivors-transmitted-trauma, accessed on 28 September 2016.

Houlihan, J., Kropp, T., Wiles, R., Gray, S., and Campbell, C. (2005) *Body Burden. The Pollution in Newborns*. Washington, DC: Environmental Working Group. Available at www.changelingaspects.com/PDF/bodyburden2_final-r3.pdf, accessed on 28 September 2016.

Lake, F. (1978) *Theological Issues in Mental Health in India*. Nottingham: Clinical Theological Association.

Maiden, A.H. and Farwell, E. (1997) *The Tibetan Art of Parenting. From Before Conception Through Early Childhood*. Boston, MA: Wisdom Publications.

Maret, S.M. (1997) *The Prenatal Person. Frank Lake's Maternal-Fetal Distress Syndrome*. Lanham, MD: University Press of America.

Montagu, A. (1965) *Life Before Birth*. New York: New American Library.

Moss, R. (1987) 'Frank Lake's Maternal-Fetal Distress Syndrome: Clinical and Theoretical Considerations.' In T.R. Verny (ed.) *Pre and Perinatal Psychology. An Introduction.* New York: Human Sciences Press.

Odent, M. (1986) *Primal Health. A Blueprint for our Survival.* London: Century.

Reich, W. (1942) *The Function of the Orgasm.* New York: Orgone Institute Press.

Somé, S. (2009) *Welcoming Spirit Home. Ancient African Teachings to Celebrate Children and Community.* Sacramento, CA: Healing Wisdom Well, Ancestors Wisdom Spring.

Terry, K. (2011) *Umbilical Affect.* Institute of Pre- and Perinatal Education.

Upledger, J. (1990) *SomatoEmotional Release and Beyond.* Palm Beach, FL: UI Publishing.

CHAPTER 7

HOW THERAPISTS CAN UNDERSTAND AND HELP WITH THE IMPLICATIONS OF WIDER FAMILY DYNAMICS

David Haas

Introduction

My initial introduction to the pre- and perinatal (PPN) therapy field was in the early 1990s while I was training as a polarity therapist. One of my trainers, Stephan Schorr Kohn, suggested that I investigate the effects of anaesthesia and analgesics in relation to Polarity Therapy for the unborn child. Stephan had been working with psychotherapist William Emerson, who specialized in psychotherapy and regression therapy for infants, children and adults. My interest in PPN continued to grow initially with Emerson and then primarily with the work of Ray Castellino. I began to work with Ray in 1996 and have continued to explore and deepen my understanding of this work with the same passion that originally drew me into this field. Ray Castellino initially practised as a chiropractor, and both a polarity and craniosacral therapist. He had studied with Emerson prior to developing his own form of PPN therapy, which included creating the BEBA[1] clinic with Wendy Anne McCarty.

---

1   BEBA (Building and Enhancing, Bonding and Attachment). In 1993 Ray Castellino and Wendy Anne McCarty opened the doors of the BEBA, a non-profit clinic, to research and work with families and their babies in the pre- and perinatal field. They co-facilitated and recorded the sessions for five years with the intention to understand what babies were showing in their sessions. See www.beba.org.

Pre- and perinatal therapy

The field of pre- and perinatal therapy can be argued to have begun with the work of Otto Rank, a student of Freud. In more recent years there has been an expansion in research and the development of therapies to support both the understanding and healing of the effects of early life trauma.

Some of the researchers who have contributed to our current understanding in this field include Frank Lake and Donald Winnicott. Winnicott brought in the concept of the 'good enough mother' (discussed later) and the importance of support in therapeutic approaches. John Bowlby brought attention to the importance of maintaining the parental bond with the infant by his research into the separation of infants from their parents when admitted to hospital. He worked together with Mary Ainsworth, who developed the Strange Situation study (see Chapter 4). As a result, the theory of secure/insecure attachment emerged and the theory of disorganized attachment was added following research by Mary Maine. Stanislov Grof developed the concept of basic perinatal matrices as well as that of condensed experiences or COEX.[2] More recent pioneers include Thomas Verney, David Chamberlain, Joseph Chilton Pearce, William Emerson, Ray Castellino and Wendy Anne McCarty. This list is far from complete and continues to grow as interest in the pre- and perinatal field expands.

For the purpose of Chapters 7 and 8 we will be focusing on the pre- and perinatal therapy work of Ray Castellino, as it brings together a method of working with and integrating the psychological and emotional imprinting that happens in early life. This approach combines working with both psychological approaches and body-based therapies.

In the beginning

I suggest that life is about relationships, whether that be intimate, family, social or work relationships. Sometimes relationships flow easily but at other times they can be a struggle.

---

2   'A COEX system consists of emotionally charged memories from different periods of our life that resemble each other in the quality of emotion or physical sensation that they share. Each COEX has a basic theme that permeates all its layers and represents their common denominator. The individual layers then contain variations on this basic theme that occurred at different periods of the person's life' (Grof 2007).

A therapeutic relationship differs fundamentally from other relationships in that it is a confidential and safe space where the client does not have to worry about taking care of the therapist. It is a relationship where the therapist holds a place of *welcome* for his client; in that place to be with his client as he or she is. In most instances, the therapist does not know the client's friends and family so he will only perceive these relationships as his client describes them. Some therapists, such as psychotherapists, are also trained and supported to recognize transference and counter-transference. I have included more information about this later in the chapter.

It might seem controversial to say this, but our earliest relationships develop within the womb. Many practitioners using hypnosis and various forms of pre- and perinatal therapy have discovered that the foetus is conscious both in the womb and during the birth process.

Michael Gabriel (1992, p.21)[3] writes about his experience: 'What proof do we have 'that prenatal memories are real or that infants who are still in the womb are responsive to their experiences'. In common with my own and colleagues' experiences, Gabriel shares how, when his clients check back with their parents, or others who would know the historical facts, their prenatal or birth experience is accurate: that the only way they would know about the event(s) is by experiencing them prior to birth.

Within Ray Castellino's framework we work with individuals, couples and families and within what are termed Womb Surround Process Workshops. These provide a safe space to explore the deep and rich feelings connected with the very early relationship formed in the womb. Speaking of this prenatal time, even before the body begins to form, Castellino suggests: 'We think consciousness is there. Our Soul pre-exists the body. The body itself is a vehicle for the expression of that Soul' (Castellino 2015b).

In the early days of our development in the womb, we are one with our mother, connected to nutrition, hormones and oxygen through our umbilical cord. We have limited ability to perceive our mother as separate – different – from our self: in effect we are merged in terms of our perception. We grow, displacing the amniotic fluid until we fill the space, indicating to our mother our readiness for moving to the world outside. Sometimes this transition occurs solely in relationship to our mother. At other times lifesaving, external help is provided, such as forceps, vacuum extraction (Ventouse) or

---

3   Note that all references in this chapter are listed at the end of Chapter 8.

Caesarean section. The use of various analgesics and anaesthetics may also be part of this experience.

We arrive into a new world, into what had previously been on the outside. The light is different, as are the sounds. We begin a new way to relate to our mother and father, as well as relating to our larger surround: our family, relatives and so on. Not only have we changed how we see our family, but we are also transforming how we receive nutrients and oxygen. A rapid transition within our heart allows our lungs to function – to breathe and exhale air. With this change we can now communicate by ourselves to the world around us through sound. We can hear, and express our feelings and needs through the medium of air. Our senses now also function through air rather than fluid. It is a time of huge change.

How we perceive these changes depends on our relationship with our primary carers. This relationship can be affected in turn by our primary carers' own history, especially their own early life experiences. As we will see, stress, whether it arises out of present-day events, or is generated as a result of *reliving* events from our history, can affect our ability to form and maintain relationships, particularly in early life.

The role of stress

In order to consider what trauma is, let's first consider stress. Stress occurs in the body as the result of external or internal stressors. It affects the body's ability to remain in homeostasis – in balance. Figure 7.1 provides an overview of the stress response. The information provided in the schematic and in the description below is taken mainly from Gerhardt (2015, pp.75–88) and Van der Kolk (2014, pp.60–63).

Figure 7.2 shows the organs of the HPA axis in their relative positions.

There are two ways the body monitors and responds to stress: the amygdala, which is associated with rapid response to danger, and the frontal lobes of the brain that take a slightly more considered approach. The amygdala forms early in our development. Gerhardt, quoting Buss *et al.* (2012), advises that 'all the main amygdala structure is formed by week 15 of the pregnancy'.

In the understanding of some, the amygdala is considered responsible for fear detection. According to the neuroscientist LeDoux (2015), the premise that the amygdala is considered to be responsible for fear detection is just an idea. It is not based on a 'scientific finding'. LeDoux, who has been studying the amygdala for more than 30 years, seeks to correct this misunderstanding. He writes that the amygdala 'is responsible for detecting and responding to threats, and only contributes to feelings of fear indirectly'. His hypothesis 'is that the feeling of "fear" results when the outcome of these various processes (attention, perception, memory, arousal) coalesce in consciousness and compel one to feel "fear"' (2015).

The amygdala receives input from the thalamus, an area of the brain responsible for collecting sensory information, and determines if there is a danger or a threat to our survival. If there is, then the sympathetic nervous system is triggered to initiate the fight/flight response. The amygdala also triggers the hypothalamus, which then initiates the production of the stress hormone, cortisol. This is through what is called the Hypothalamus–Pituitary–Adrenal axis – commonly referred to as the HPA axis. The result of cortisol being produced affects, amongst other things, our ability to heal, learn and relax. It also causes our body to transform stored energy into a form ready to be used. This supports the fight/flight part of the autonomic nervous system's response to a perceived or real threat to survival. The HPA axis routing to provide the extra energy takes longer than the activation of the initial fight/flight response.

The slower layer of monitoring and response to the thalamus information comes from the hippocampus, anterior cingulate and the prefrontal medial cortex. Van der Kolk calls this 'the rational brain, for a conscious and much more refined interpretation'. Where there is sufficient resilience in this part of the brain to the stress response, we can interpret the situation for what it is and effectively override the amygdala's reaction. The parts of the brain can continue to function in an integrated, yet differentiated way, allowing us to remain responsive rather than reactive.

Gerhardt refers to research that indicates that in some ways a little or moderate stress may be beneficial for the baby. It is when stress becomes more intense or chronic that it can create problems. We know from our own experience as adults what stress feels like and what it does to us. However, for babies it is probably somewhat different, or at least the focus of it is. As you will read later in this chapter, resources[4] are an important factor in dealing with stress and trauma, and as Gerhardt explains:

---

4   A resource is something which is supportive of us in a way that gives us greater capacity to deal with challenges. It can be emotional, mental or associated with our spiritual well-being. As such, it can be internal or external to us. I explain this further later in the chapter.

Babies' resources are so limited that they cannot keep themselves alive, so it is very stressful for them if the mother is not there or does not respond quickly… Without the parent's help, they could in fact die.

We may feel that stress within the parent–baby dyad is a problem. As we will see within Chapters 7 and 8, stress does affect our ability to relate. However, there is an importance for baby to be able to stress her parents. Gerhardt points out that when the baby is distressed, her cries 'create stress for the parent in turn, cutting through the parent's dangerous inattention, to ensure a response – and with it the baby's survival'.

Having too much of something and/or for too long can create challenges. Too much cortisol is a case in point. Gerhardt writes about cortisol that 'it can have some very unhelpful side effects if the stress is not resolved or the stress response cycle is not working properly and the production of cortisol continues'. One example she gives is the effect on the hippocampus.

Just like any other control system, some form of feedback is necessary to ensure the system, in this case the cortisol creation system, remains within certain limits. This feedback is provided to the hypothalamus by the hippocampus cortisol receptors that monitor the cortisol level. When the correct level of cortisol in the system is reached, the hippocampus signals the hypothalamus, which in turn stops the release of cortisol. Gerhardt explains that where babies have been exposed to too much stress there is a reduction in these 'hippocampal cortisol receptors'.[5] This results in a breakdown of the feedback loop to the hypothalamus, leading to excess cortisol. Remember that the action of cortisol, at least in part, affects our ability to learn, heal and relax. Gerhardt writes that:

When high levels of cortisol persist, they can shrink and reduce connections in the orbitofrontal cortex,[6] and the medial prefrontal cortex, including the anterior cingulate[7] – making them less effective in managing the more urgent reactions generated by the amygdala.

---

5   Gerhardt refers to McEwen *et al.* (2012) and Caldji, Diorio and Meaney (2000).
6   Gerhardt quoting from Hanson *et al.* (2010).
7   Gerhardt quoting from Radley and Morrison (2005).

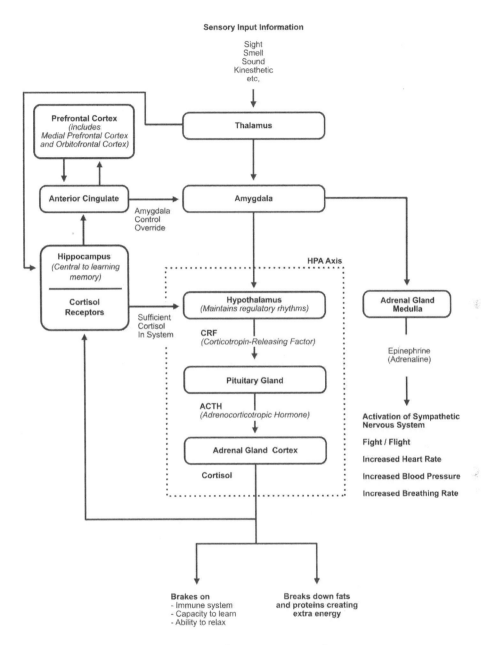

Figure 7.1 The stress response cycle

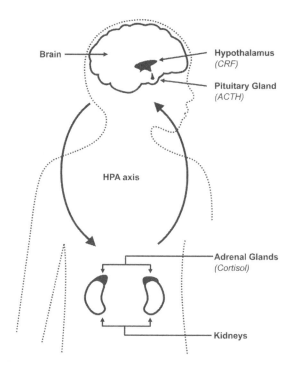

Figure 7.2 Organs of the HPA axis in their relative physical positions

There is another, more positive side to this proverbial coin. As part of the research into the loss of hippocampal cortisol receptors, Gerhardt also mentions that 'babies who are touched and held a great deal have an abundance of cortisol receptors in the hippocampus as adults'.

Within these chapters, we will see how our ability to self-regulate and deal with stressful situations comes from the support of our parents and other primary carers. They help us in infancy in modelling our response to stress – our ability to self-regulate. The importance of this is named by Gerhardt (2015) as: …the effectiveness of the stress response system is affected by how much early stress it has to deal with, and how well the system is helped to recover.

Regarding prenatal stress and its effect in early life post-birth, Gerhardt (2015) refers to research from DiPietro *et al.* (2006). The activity of a 'special enzyme in the placenta' normally blocks the passage of the stress hormone cortisol from reaching the foetus. The problem arises where the mother is in situations where she feels out of control: situations such as domestic violence and 'feeling *compelled* to work long hours'. Over a period of time, these *stressors* can cause a reduction in the special enzyme activity. The outcome is that the foetus is thereby affected by the mother's stress. Gerhardt cites further research that where babies have been in this situation they 'are born more irritable and prone to crying'. Later in this chapter we also refer to the work by Rachel Yehuda on the effect of post-traumatic stress disorder (PTSD).

The autonomic nervous system and the development of trauma

Historical view of the autonomic nervous system

Historically the autonomic nervous system (ANS) has been described as having two main components: the sympathetic and the parasympathetic branches. Within this model, the natural function is for the nervous system to self-regulate – flowing from sympathetic arousal to parasympathetic braking.

The sympathetic branch is responsible for both arousal, building energy for actions, and for reacting to threats of survival with the *fight–flight* response. The parasympathetic provides a space for healing, digestion and relaxation. The parasympathetic is also responsible for the *freeze* state that follows on when the fight–flight response is ineffective in meeting the survival needs of the individual.

In terms of early life development, Siegel (2012, p.311) writes that:

> …the sympathetic branch's development predominates during the first year of life. The parasympathetic branch comes online in the second year. This timing is helpful because as the infant becomes ambulatory, it is important to have some way in which the primary emotional states mediated by the sympathetic branch – interest/excitement and enjoyment/joy – can be modulated in order to inhibit potentially dangerous behaviours.[8]

As adults, children and babies, when we are well resourced, we are better able to process and integrate input from the world around us while remaining in relationship. Within this zone the autonomic nervous system is said to be in balance. There is a natural flow between sympathetic arousal and then parasympathetic settling (Figure 7.3): it is operating in what has been called the *functional range* by Castellino, the *window of tolerance* (Siegel 2012, pp.281–286), or the *range of resiliency* by Levine. It is also referenced

---

8   Siegel is quoting Panksepp (1998, 2009, 2010) and Panksepp and Biven (2012) here.

by Ogden, Minton and Pain (2006, p.27) as the *optimal arousal zone*.[9]
Castellino explains that the functional range 'is the range where we can have
presence and the presence is directly related to the Blueprint'.[10] (Castellino,
Jackson and Blanco, 2013–2017) It is a place of health: a place to process
and integrate traumatic experiences. Within this space, we function well.

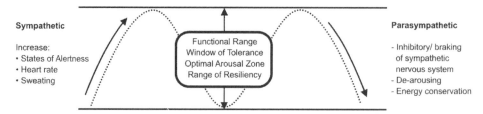

Figure 7.3 Natural cycling of the ANS showing the functional range and window of tolerance

For each person, and in different circumstances, the width of the window
can vary. It is dependent on what is happening in the current moment, as
well as based on our history, particularly our early history. I agree with
my Swiss friend and colleague, psychotherapist and PPN therapist Klaus
Käppeli, that the width of the window is also very dependent on how well
a baby is securely attached at the beginning of her life. Secure bonding
and attachment creates self-confidence and trust that widens the window
of tolerance. Ongoing research is showing that how our parents adapted to
their environment can be transferred to their children, possibly over several
more generations. There is more on this later in the chapter.

Support, particularly layers of support, and feeling safe are types of resource
that can help individuals remain in the window of tolerance and widen it.
On the other hand, physical exhaustion and hunger may, according to Siegel
(2012, p.283), 'also markedly restrict individuals' windows of tolerance and
make them more vulnerable to irritability and "emotional outbursts"'. In other
words, the ability for healthy functioning becomes challenged.

Within the window of tolerance or functional range, we are in the natural
cycling, or ebb and flow, of the autonomic nervous system, or what is termed
the optimal arousal zone. Outside of this zone we move into hyperarousal,
characterized by an increase of sympathetic branch symptoms such as fight
and flight. Where the conditions are such that fight or flight are unachievable

---

9   Ogden reference taken from Wilbarger and Wilbarger (1997).
10   The Blueprint is a term taken from Polarity Therapy. This form of energy is perceived to be
     present prior to conception. More detail is provided later in this chapter.

in that moment, parasympathetic braking is applied and we shift into the hypoarousal state: that of the energy-conserving, loss of vagal tone, freeze and dissociative states.

Let us consider this in some more detail. Initially the autonomic nervous system is cycling naturally within the window of tolerance. Something changes in our perception: something within our sensory mechanism perceives a reduction in our safety – a possible threat. The body's autonomic nervous system's response is to shift into the *alarm* state. That is, into the early stages of the sympathetic branch arousal. If the threat goes away, then there is a return to settling. If the threat continues, the arousal level increases, creating the energy necessary for fight or flight. In either case, when we have fought or run away, the arousal energy is dissipated and we return to normal life. This is what happens with animals in the wild. If we are unable to fight or run (or perceive this to be the case) the parasympathetic *brake* is applied, taking us into parasympathetic shock or what is more commonly referred to as the *freeze* state. Levine and Frederick (1997, pp.15–16) say of this state:

> The stone-still animal is not pretending to be dead. It has instinctively entered an altered state of consciousness shared by all mammals when death appears imminent.

They further write that it is believed animals in the wild use this freeze or immobility response of the nervous system to 'play dead' and in so doing so survive their predator. A second reason is that in this altered state the animal will not experience pain. However, within this state, the nervous system still contains this explosive arousal energy created to escape the threat. Animals that escape will then shake, run or jump to dissipate the energy and return to the nervous system operating in its normal functional range: This is natural and normal. But when this discharge is prevented, we are left with a traumatic imprint. Trauma imprints will be discussed in more detail later in the chapter. According to Levine and Kline (2007, pp.13–14), this issue is more likely to occur with humans rather than animals due in part to humans having the ability to think and self-judge, thereby preventing the natural return to homeostasis.

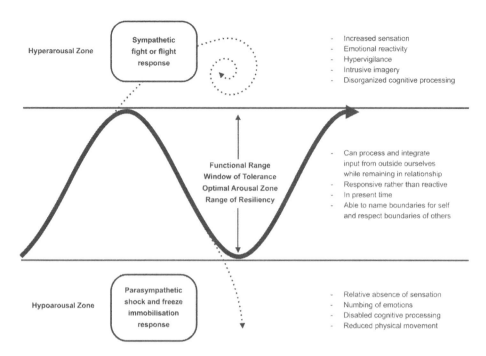

Figure 7.4 Window of tolerance with the autonomic nervous system and arousal states

Figure 7.4 was developed from the work of many people over the years. Those that we are aware of include Levine, Anna Chitty,[11] Castellino and Ogden *et al.* (2006). It shows the effect of overwhelm causing an acceleration out of the window of tolerance into a vortex and then with the application of the parasympathetic brake dropping into the freeze/dissociative states. The negative result of the creation of the trauma imprint is a persistent narrowing of the functional range – the window of tolerance. When we are able to sit within the window of tolerance we are in a responsive state and are reactive either side of it. This narrowing reduces the opportunity to be in a relational, responsive state. To be able to be present in relationship and attuned with another person we need to be within the window of tolerance. This has particular ramifications for working with babies and children.

Gerhardt (2015, p.65) points out how much a child depends 'on the parent for regulation of his states, whether physiological or psychological'. The greater the window of tolerance in the adult means that she has greater ability to self-regulate in more challenging conditions. I suggest that the outcome of this supports the child's nervous system to also develop a broader

---

11   Anna Chitty is the director of the Biodynamic Craniosacral Therapy foundation programme and advanced courses at the Colorado School of Energy Studies.

window of tolerance and thereby be more available for secure attachment and all the benefits that brings.

The Polyvagal Theory of the nervous system

The Polyvagal Theory was developed by Dr Stephen Porges as a result of his extensive studies into the evolutionary development of our autonomic nervous system. In an interview (Porges 2013), he explains his discovery that took him on the route to develop the Polyvagal Theory. It was that the historical understanding of the relationship between the sympathetic and parasympathetic nervous systems created a paradox in relation to the vagus nerve. He found that the vagus nerve was serving in both a protective form and in a lethal form. In his research with newborns he measured vagal activity in terms of heart rate response. He found that 'newborns had good clinical outcomes if they had a lot of this vagal activity, which is represented in a rhythmic heart rate modulation.' This 'is called respiratory sinus arrhythmia and he describes it as 'the heart rate is going up and down with breathing.' However, it appeared that the vagus nerve can also cause bradycardia and apnoea,[12] which is life-threatening for many preterm infants.

The outcome was his discovery of two vagal systems, one for each side of this paradox. Each of these vagus nerves arises out of different parts of the brain. One is myelinated and the other is not. The former, the *new mammalian vagus* as he calls it, is linked to the area of the brainstem that 'regulates the muscles of the face and head'. This vagal nerve forms the basis for what he defines as the *social engagement system*;[13] together with the sympathetic and the unmyelinated vagal circuit they form the hierarchical autonomic nervous system. This is the concept of the Polyvagal Theory.

Porges (2013) also coined the term *neuroception*. 'It is detection without awareness. It as a neural circuit that evaluates risk in the environment from a variety of clues'. So if our perception of the situation is low risk or safe, neuroception places us in the social engagement system, which he sees as

---

12 Infant apnoea is where breathing stops, with one or more of these characteristics:
    Lasting more than 20 seconds.
    The baby's colour may change to pale, purplish or blue.
    Slowing of the heart rate, known as a bradycardia.
13 Porges (2011, Figure 3.1) shows the social engagement system overview. It involves the cranial nerves V, VII, IX, X and XI, which involve muscles of mastication, middle ear and facial, as well as the larynx, pharynx, head turning, bronchi and heart.

the *preamble to attachment*: it is the place that supports developing secure attachment. When we cannot get our needs met, or we perceive increased risk and danger, neuroception shifts us to the sympathetic nervous system response. We are into the option of fight or flight. As in the historic mode of the autonomic nervous system, when that option fails to support survival, we shift into the ancient unmyelinated vagal circuit into the freeze and shut down system.

Porges explains that being in a physiological state that supports fight/ flight does not support social behaviour, and 'If we are in a physiological state that is shutting down, we are, functionally, immune to social interaction'. Not good news for supporting the development of secure attachment!

Siegel (2010, p.23) adds that with the inability to activate the social engagement system, we are also unable to 'access a *self-engagement system*'. We move out of being present and 'become removed, alone, and paralysed'.

In relation to maladaptive reactions in certain situations, such as pounding heart, sweating hands and fear of passing out, Porges (2013) expects that:

> …as more research is conducted we will probably learn that early experiences play an important role in changing the threshold or vulnerability to express these apparently maladaptive reactions. If we are protected with the newer vagal circuit, we do fine. However, if we lose regulation of this newer vagal circuit, we become, in a sense, basically defensive fight–flight machines.

Figure 7.5 shows the arousal states in relation to the hierarchical process proposed by the Polyvagal Theory.

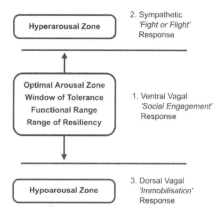

Figure 7.5 The correlation of the three arousal zones and the polyvagal hierarchy (Ogden et al. 2006, Figure 2.2), with minor modifications

Trauma

In recent years much has been written about trauma and how it might be healed. There is a growing shift amongst psychotherapists from working purely with cognitive processes to including the somatic experience – working with the autonomic and social nervous systems.

So what is trauma? Trauma results from our body's inability to process an event. It occurs when we don't have the capacity or resources to digest and integrate the event. Figure 7.6 is a simplified schematic of this process. This lack of capacity or resources explains why one person may be traumatized by an event while another is not. Trauma is in effect what is left over, what remains from an overwhelming event. It is an imprint. Levine and Kline (2007, p.4) write that 'trauma is not in the event itself; rather, trauma resides in the nervous system'.

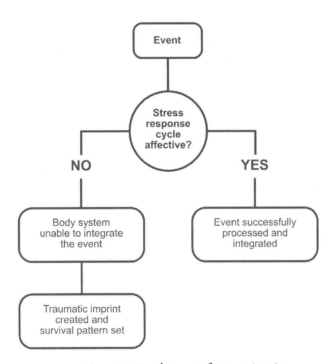

Figure 7.6 Development of trauma imprints

Earlier in the chapter I wrote about the research of DiPietro *et al.* (2006) and the cortisol blocking enzyme. While the HPA and stress response systems are not available to the prenate, the prenate is relying on her mother's stress response system to deal with overwhelm. I suggest that where her mother cannot integrate the event, leading to the trauma imprint for herself, this may well affect her foetus.

The foetus and baby are dependent on the connection with their mother and other primary carers to provide the resources necessary to integrate stressful situations. Where that connection may disappear, for example when general anaesthesia is used during birth, then this may create trauma imprints.

Van der Kolk (2014, p.43) makes the very powerful statement:

All trauma is preverbal.

He clarifies this in a further statement:

Trauma by nature drives us to the edge of comprehension, cutting us off from language based on common experience or an imaginable past.

Van der Kolk explains how these statements, in part, arise from the discovery of what happens to a region of the brain called Broca's area when a trauma imprint is being relived. This area is one of the speech centres of the brain. The experiment utilized a tape-recording of a script that had been prepared with each participant that related to the traumatic event in their history. They played the tape to the participant while they were in the fMRI (functional Magnetic Resonance Imaging) scanner. They noticed that while the participant re-experienced the sensations and emotions of the trauma imprint, Broca's area went offline. 'Without a functioning Broca's area you cannot put your thoughts and feelings into words.' (Van der Kolk 2014)

We have examined the different responses to a traumatic event: fight or flight, or where that fails, the move into the freeze or dissociated state. The possibility for adults to escape a traumatic event by running or fighting does not exist in early life. At this stage of development, the infant is dependent on his attachment figure, in other words his parent or other primary carer, for protection and/or to escape the situation. Where this does not work, the baby's body system has to mobilize its own form of protection. One reaction to the overwhelming event is dissociation. Gerhardt (2015, p.188) describes it as 'a crude attempt to cut off contact with other people who might generate further (unpleasant) sympathetic nervous system arousal'.

There is another aspect that is particular to babies and children. Where a situation arises that feels unsafe or overwhelming, they will want to move close enough to their primary carers to feel safe. The challenge arises where the attachment figure is also the cause of the fear – the lack of safety. As they depend on their primary carers for their survival, it creates a *double bind* imprint: whichever way the child goes does not provide the safety she needs.

It is important to remember that we see trauma as our reaction to an event from the outside that was too much for us to integrate. It is the outcome of how we did our best in certain circumstances and certain situations. We found a way through to survive, even if it resulted in a fragmentation in our psyche. We developed patterns of behaviour and adapted to survive. For the healing process to begin we need to perceive and accept, with love and support, that fragmented part of our younger self. She is identified with the survival pattern, and if we attempt to just push the pattern away, or *get rid of it*, we believe that our younger self will feel we are trying to get rid of her. She will respond in the only way she knows how: with her survival response.

Imprints

Our brain records the events and sequences in both implicit and explicit memory. Implicit memory is considered a nonverbal memory and includes feelings and sensations, whereas explicit memory provides factual and autobiographical aspects. Implicit memory is with us in the beginning, whereas semantic memory 'becomes available at around a year and a half of age, and autobiographical memory, which begins to develop some time after the second birthday' (Siegel and Hartzell 2003, p.23). According to Siegel (2010, p.64), 'For many of us, explicit memory is not available in any continuous way for the time before we were about five years of age – or even 3, or a year and a half.' When both the explicit and implicit memories are online, we can put words to feelings and create a coherent historical narrative.

Before the explicit memory is mature, or when we have a challenging experience that we are unable to integrate, such as a traumatic experience, we are left with only the implicit memory recording feelings and sensations. In other words we are left with only the feelings and sensations related to the traumatic event but with no sense of time. Van der Kolk (2014, p.176) explains:

> Under ordinary conditions these two memory systems – rational and emotional – collaborate to produce an integrated response. But high arousal not only changes the balance between them but also disconnects other brain areas necessary for the proper storage and integration of incoming

information, such as the hippocampus and the thalamus. As a result, the imprints of traumatic experiences are organized not as coherent logical narratives but in fragmented sensory and emotional traces: images, sounds, and physical sensations.

When historic trauma memories are recalled, we experience the feelings and sensations without the story. With no ability to determine when they occurred, they will feel to us as if they are related to the present.

You may have noticed when you have reacted to an event, such as a statement from someone else, in a way that is out of context. You may even be aware of watching yourself react, whilst wondering why you are behaving this way. This is usually an indication that we are accessing a historic event and reacting as if this event was happening today.

To recap, an imprint is what remains with us following an event. It is not who we are, rather it has formed on our nervous system. It does not change who we are, yet it affects how we are within the world. It affects how we respond to the environment around us. As Porges (2013) points out, 'it is the response [to the environmental challenge], and not the traumatic event, that is critical'.

An analogy of an imprint would be to imagine taking a tin and filling it with warm wax. If you take a key, you can push it into the warm wax. When the wax hardens and you remove the key, an imprint of the key remains. The wax is remembering the key. Creating the imprint has not changed the constitution of the wax. We can see that if the wax is reheated, it flows to fill the space and the imprint disappears.

As we dissipate the energy of the imprint, develop the coherent narrative, and place the story in its true place in our history, we become more of the conscious being that we truly are. This is why it can be immensely useful when working with early traumatic events for clients to be able to put these imprints in a specific historical context.

Types of imprint

As part of the pre- and perinatal therapy work, we consider a variety of possible external events that can cause imprints. I have mentioned one or two of these above and include a more extensive list below that was developed by Ray Castellino. Although the list can appear focused on birth, some of the imprints fall within the prenatal period. From his work he noted the types of pattern that may arise in an individual for each of the imprints. The list is not exhaustive.

It is important to remember that just because an intervention was made or a situation occurred, such as a nuchal cord[14] or shoulder dystocia,[15] it does not mean that the individual will create a survival imprint pattern in response. If there are sufficient resources, then the event can be integrated. A primary resource for the prenate would be her mother. In turn, what helps her mother to be present are the resources she herself has – such as layers of support, which I will discuss in more detail later in the chapter. A recognized resource for premature babies is what is called Kangaroo Care. The baby is held in skin-to-skin contact with an adult – usually her parent. I will discuss more about this later in the chapter in the section on resources.

Also, let us not forget that the use of drugs and some medical procedures can be lifesaving and necessary.

- Chemical imprints[16]

  » Anaesthesia/Analgesics

  » Synthetic oxytocin (induction)

  » Recreational drugs such as:

    - Alcohol

    - Nicotine

    - Cocaine

    - Marijuana

    - Caffeine.

---

14 Nuchal cord is where the umbilical cord is wrapped around the baby's neck.

15 Shoulder dystocia is where in labour the baby's head has been delivered and one of the baby's shoulders becomes stuck behind her mother's pubic bone.

16 Castellino advised that 'The effect of shock and trauma imprints (often specifically drug imprints) causes the sympathetic [nervous system] wave to accelerate off the top of the curve, whilst causing the parasympathetic [nervous system] wave to drop off the bottom of the curve into shock and freeze' (Castellino *et al.* 2013–2017, p.47). This is shown in Figure 7.4.

- Surgical and mechanical imprints[17]

  » Forceps

  » Ventouse (vacuum extraction)

  » Caesarean section

  » Circumcision.

- Other imprints

  » Ultrasound

  » Amniocentesis

  » Twin loss[18]

  » Twin dynamics[19]

  » Double bind or paradoxical[20]

  » Ancestral.

---

17 Gerhardt (2015, p.88) quoting Gunnar *et al.* (1985a, 1985b): 'In newborn babies, the stress response can be generated by physical danger such as a forceps delivery or circumcision.'

18 While twin loss can occur at any time, it is particularly important to consider the outcome when it occurs in utero, especially early on in the pregnancy. Emerson (1996) states: 'embryologists conclude that many conceptions involved the death of one or more twins, usually prior to or during implantation, although some happen after implantation'. Chamberlain (2006) writes of his discovery of babies having 'an innate sense of self, memory, intelligence, virtue, awareness, and knowing'. He continues about the babies being capable of 'storing out-of-body experiences and even near-death experiences in response to abortion attempts and the loss of a twin in utero'.

19 Emerson (1996) writes about several common dynamics that can be experienced where there has been a twin loss. He writes of how these experiences can affect life after birth. Within his description he includes challenges in the ability to bond – 'unarticulated feelings that loss will happen again' – as well as 'pervasive insecurity' and 'over compliance' amongst other possible outcomes.
    With the loss of a twin as described above, the twin that survives is undifferentiated from the twin that died. This is the twin dynamic. They were/are merged. Castellino explains this as: 'There is no feeling of difference between the twin that leaves and me. [I] don't know if I left or stayed.' Castellino *et al.* 2013–2017) This creates a paradox, and as Castellino goes on to say: 'That is the dilemma of the *lost* twin.' The surviving twin does not know if I left or stayed. He goes on to say: 'That relationship [between the twins] often feels closer, more prominent than any other earthly relationship we have.'

20 Double binds arise out of the dynamic of 'whichever way I choose there is not a good solution'. An example is a child in a setting with his parent. He needs to be with his parent for safety and security, yet his parent in the disorganized attachment setting is the cause of the danger. There is an inner to and fro, but because this can be quite fast, it can paradoxically feel a very *stuck* place.

Umbilical affect forms part of the list of imprints and is discussed in more depth in Chapter 6. This type of imprint can be caused by chemical, hormonal and/or surgical factors.

Each of the above has its own specific or *signature* imprint(s). For example, Castellino describes the effect that it is easy to lose orientation when anaesthesia has been used. While alcohol is 'like a shade slowly pulling down over a window' or 'heaviness and tiredness to keep awake'.

Some drugs have the effect of creating an imprint of slowing down and others of speeding up. Some create a sense of dissociation whilst others create loss of feeling.

For baby, ancestral imprints arise from her parent's history and generationally back to include grandparents, great-grandparents and so on. It becomes more complex where there have been family splits and then new relationships formed. It is especially complex in cases of adoption, where there are two completely separate family systems with their own historic imprints.

The effect of ancestral trauma affecting future generations is being researched in the field of neuroscience: particularly in the field of epigenetics. In a radio interview, Yehuda (2015) speaks about being able to acknowledge that 'trauma effects last. They endure, they don't all go away. Epigenetics allow us to extend it to generational.'

Yehuda and her colleagues carried out their research by initially establishing a clinic for holocaust survivors and studying their children. Additionally, they also studied the children of pregnant women who survived the 9/11 attack on the World Trade Center in New York. The children of the holocaust survivors shared that they felt 'traumatised by witnessing the symptoms of their parents'. They felt the expectations placed on them – things that they would have to achieve in order to give meaning to those who died. Also that they had 'difficulty in any kind of a separation circumstance' such as divorce and separating from their parents.

Yehuda explains in the interview that there are two ways to influence the next generation. One is through an *epigenetic mark* on your gene, which gets transmitted to the next generation during cell division. She defines that as a transmitted change and concludes with her colleagues (Yehuda *et al.* 2015) that:

This is the first demonstration of an association of pre-conception parental trauma with epigenetic alterations that is evident in both exposed parent and offspring, providing potential insight into how severe psychophysiological trauma can have intergenerational effects.

The other form of change that Yehuda mentions in the radio interview (2015) is where a set of circumstances are created at conception, post-conception or in utero where the foetus 'is *forced* to make an adaptation[21] to those circumstances'.

Imprints and adaptations affect us and how we relate in the world. At first glance, it can appear that they always have a negative outcome. However, some imprints and adaptations can still be useful in life. What is important is for the shock energy (the energy that was initially created as part of the fight–flight mechanism and could not be naturally discharged) to be dissipated sufficiently so that we can choose whether to use the imprint – the survival strategy – or not.

It is important to remember, as mentioned earlier in this chapter, that the creation of a traumatic imprint depends on the resources available to the individual. With sufficient resources it is considered possible to integrate the event.

Sequences

When a number of imprints follow on from each other, a sequence is created. An example of a sequence is being born. Wilks (2015, p.180) writes of the stages of vaginal birth being defined in traditional midwifery as:

1. Onset of labour to complete dilation of the cervix

2. Birth of the baby

3. Delivery of the placenta.

In the 1990s, William Emerson, Ray Castellino and Franklyn Sills chose to consider the journey from the inside out, rather than the traditional midwifery perspective of outside in. In other words, looking from the baby's perspective. Castellino (2015a) describes it thus:

---

21   Adaptation is defined as 'a feature of an organism's structure, physiology, or behaviour that solves a problem in its life or helps it to pass on genes to the next generation' (Colman 2015).

The birth stages according to Emerson are based on what the baby has to do to negotiate his/her way through its mother's pelvic passage as a cranial (head first) vaginal birth:

Stage one	Inlet dynamics	Baby's head engages the pelvic inlet
Stage two	Mid-pelvic dynamics	The baby's head negotiates the mid-pelvis, passing zero station of the ischial spines
Stage three	Outlet dynamics	Baby's head is born and restitutes
Stage four	Baby's shoulders and body are born.	Routine medical interventions are done including the cutting of the umbilical cord

Castellino goes on to reflect how imprints during the developmental stages of preconception through pregnancy are 'recapitulated' through the stages of the birth process. The inability to differentiate history from present-day life can create difficulties in all forms of relationship and in our ability to do what we really want in our lives. As already mentioned, let us not forget that some of these imprints or patterns can be useful in our lives. They can be what are perceived as strengths. The issue is more about having choice. I suggest that the energy held in the trauma imprint is such that it *drives* the survival pattern. Being a survival pattern, it is about reacting to survive rather than responding to an event. This means that when in survival mode we have less conscious choice in our lives.

To support healing, we need to be able to connect with the implicit memory imprint and to find a coherent narrative which supports us to establish a bridge between the past and the present. In the process of creating the coherent narrative we also are integrating between the left and right brain. Castellino feels that 'the sense organ that gives us the window between now and then is the eyes' Castellino *et al.* (2013–2017). By pausing and looking around where we are and who we are with, we are reorienting to the present day, to present time. We can hopefully perceive today, with those around us in this space, that we are safe. In other words, our eyes help us to orient to present time and so support us to differentiate from our historic implicit imprints.

An example of orientating to present time by differentiating layers of history comes from an interview that independent midwife Mary Jackson (Jackson 2015) gave on this subject: it includes a summary of the effect of early life imprints and sequences. Mary provided a case history of how a pregnant mother's own birthing history affected the birth of her children. She supported the mother to differentiate her own history and thereby to develop a coherent narrative with the feelings and sensations from her own birth.

She tells the story of a mum who was strongly impacted when she was being born. Her birth went very fast, and the imprint that stayed with her was a fear of moving too quickly: the speed of labour was faster than she could integrate. When this mum was having her own first baby she got to 8 cm diameter and the labour sped up so quickly that it was terrifying for her. In her second labour it was also pretty fast from 3 cm to birth.

In her third labour there was a huge fear about hitting the place where it felt to her that it *just takes off* and feels out of control, way faster than her natural rhythm. Her fear was that she would not be able to integrate each step of the way in her labour because it was going so fast that she would end up having to integrate afterwards. This time at about 4 cm dilation she got stuck and they talked about the fear of hitting that speed-up/fast place. At this point the contractions stopped. Mary supported her to be in connection with the slower rhythm inside herself and also being able to connect with the baby in his slower rhythm. She then supported the mum to differentiate the layers that were created in her birth with her mother. She was also able to differentiate the layers around what happened with her first and second births and what she was wanting for this third birth.

When the mum became clear on the different parts of her history around dilation and speed-up with what she wanted this time, her labour restarted at a slower pace. Now that labour was proceeding at a more natural pace, she was able to integrate the process as she was going through it. The outcome was that the third labour went at a pace that she was able to integrate and thereby stay with the experience as it happened. In this way she was not having to integrate it after the fact.

Mary summarizes: 'When I remind her [the current-day mother in labour] what her history with her own mum was, she can differentiate and it supports the labour to move on and continue to birth her baby at home. So it is really useful.'

What are resources?

Resources provide a way for us to process and integrate an event, whether it is happening in the moment or due to an historic trauma imprint. With resources we can take steps and actions that we were unable to take in our earlier life – to complete the cycle of integration and have expression of our feelings and sensations that were held in the trauma imprint.

Resources can be either internal or external, or both. They might be everyday events that are simple, such as enjoying a cup of our favourite tea by oneself or with friends. Examples of internal resources could be something we can connect to within our self, a place within us that feels good, flowing and open. Remembering a time in our lives when we felt good, where we felt loved or held. Perhaps following a spiritual practice. It might be feeling good sensations within our body such as warmth or energies that are uplifting or settling.

External resources can be varied. Within the pre- and perinatal work we provide external resources to our clients in order to assist them in making sense and integrating their traumatic imprints. Some of the resources that are used in therapy are listed here and then expanded on later in this chapter:

- Support

- Attunement and harmonic resonance

- Relational tide

- Blueprint energy

- Midspace exercise

- Dynamic creative opposition exercise – being met in our power and developing tone in our body.

Certain of the core principles developed by Castellino to support the structure within our form of the pre- and perinatal therapy work are also external resources. These are described later in the chapter.

What may be a resource for one person, such as a beautiful beach holiday, may bring up challenging memories for someone who experienced a tsunami while on a beach holiday. Similarly, a special doll or family pet could be a positive resource for an infant or perhaps something frightening. Resources are unique to each of us.

Sometimes clients have difficulty connecting to a resource that appears positive. Ogden *et al.* (2006, p.208) remind us that:

> Although clients may feel they have no resources…even the most dysregulated client has used survival resources that may go unnoticed until the therapist draws attention to them.

Also the importance of assessing and establishing resources, both existing and missing, are considered to be a priority as therapy begins and develops over sessions. As the client speaks about a resource, the therapist can track him somatically to feel whether the resource is really supportive or not.

In early life we are very dependent on our primary carers to provide resources for us. It is not that we don't have resources, but in our early years we are very vulnerable to what comes in from the outside; our inner resources have yet to achieve the depth and strength that we develop as we grow into adulthood.

An example of resources provided to preterm babies is Kangaroo Care (KC). It was first introduced in Colombia, as they did not have incubators to support preterm babies. In KC the prenate is held in skin-to-skin contact with an adult who provides contact, natural body temperature and nervous system regulation. McGregor and Casey (2012)[22] advise that some of the positive outcomes of KC are 'cardio-respiratory stabilisation, increasing sleep, decreasing signs of agitation, increasing the rate of weight gain, improving thermoregulation, shortening hospital stay and functioning as analgesia'. KC might also be considered as providing support for early attachment and bonding. McGregor and Casey go on to point out how many of the bonding processes can be disrupted for many premature infants if they are separated from their mothers after birth.

We believe that during pregnancy and birth, the more the mother can develop a relationship with her baby, the more resources are available, especially during labour and birth. As you will read later on in this chapter, creating layers of support can help mothers to relax and be in relationship with their baby both in utero and in early life.

Some babies are born with their mothers having been anaesthetized. I have worked with adults who were born this way. As they have somatically revisited their birth pattern history in a therapy session, they were able to

---

22 Quoting Dodd (2005), Johnson (2005) and Ludington-Hoe and Swinth (1996).

name their experience of the *loss of connection* with their mother and the feelings and sensations that go with that loss. This occurs shortly before they touch the place in their birth where the anaesthetic reached them and they lost consciousness. With support they are able to re-pattern their original somatic experience into what they would have wanted.

Support

To receive support is not always easy. Our historical imprints can challenge our ability to be open to receive in this way. This could be because in our past the offer of support came with strings attached or perhaps an expectation to give something back. However, what we are finding in therapy work is that support is a very necessary resource. Castellino coined the phrase 'two layers of support' (Castellino 2014) as a necessary requirement for families to relax, 'let down' and deepen in themselves and so be more able to come into attunement with each other.

In this context, support forms a useful resource as it increases the capacity to integrate events that on our own would be too much, and possibly even result in trauma imprints.

As part of my presentation at a Birthlight conference in London, I presented an exercise on support with two of my colleagues, Kitty Hagenbach and Chantek McNeilage. Kitty took the role of receiving support and Chantek of providing the first layer of support. Support can be provided in different forms, but in this case it was provided as physical contact to Kitty's lower back. Wherever possible, making physical contact is done through careful negotiation. Once the first level of support was established we noted some settling; in other words, a feeling of letting down, relaxing within our bodies. I then provided the second layer of support in the same way to Chantek's lower back and the settling deepened significantly. Some of the audience members fed back to me that when the second layer of support was established they felt themselves settling. It appears that it is not just those receiving direct support that benefit!

While good support, and in particular two-layer support, is useful throughout our lives, it is especially important in early life as this is where we lay down foundations for the rest of our lives.

An example of receiving early life support comes from Mary Jackson. For a while she offered all her clients coming for midwifery support three PPN therapy sessions with Ray Castellino and herself.

How the parents were born, their own labour and birth history, can affect whether they are able to be 'present' or not at their baby's birth. This in turn can affect how labour and birth progress. Implicit memory when activated only provides sensations and feelings. As already mentioned, if during the mother's labour an implicit memory of contraction and fear from what happened in her own birth (as opposed to what is happening in present time for her baby's birth) is touched, it can affect how her baby's birth turns out. With the support provided, parents are able to relax and get some clarity around their own imprints and so be more present for each other and their baby's birth.

During this period, Mary noted that the transfer to hospital decreased from 20 per cent to 3 per cent; also that the rate of perineal tears decreased by 50 per cent and that all babies were fed from the breast.

Layers of support can be created in most situations. Figure 7.7 shows what is possible in a home birth. Note that there are additional layers available outside the home: the family and community, the birthing unit and the hospital.

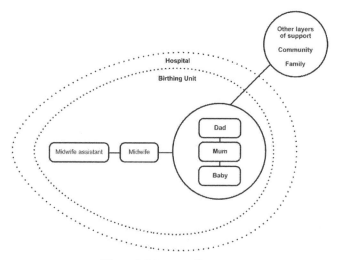

Figure 7.7 Layers of support

To demonstrate how these layers of support can be used within a mother and baby therapy session, I would like to share a typical example that is related to challenges with feeding. I will call the mother Geraldine, and the newborn, Michael.

Michael was wanting to latch on to feed and Geraldine was trying really hard to help him. By the time I arrived they had been trying for a while and were getting exhausted. The harder they tried the more exhausted they became, and in turn it became more difficult to achieve what they both so wanted: to connect, latch on and feed.

My first step was to sit and orient to present time. I generally do this by simply observing where I am in that moment, which in this case was in a room with Geraldine and Michael. I also remind myself of the date and my current age. In this way I can differentiate my own history from what is happening here in present time. This simple process supports me in settling deeper into myself and being more available to be in relationship with the family. The Midspace exercise, which I expand on below in the section on attunement, resonance and harmonic resonance, can be very useful in supporting settling and centring.

When working therapeutically, it is very important not to go in with the intention to *fix* anything in order to achieve an outcome. All that does is to add another layer to the existing confusion and activation. It is also easy to focus too narrowly on what is happening. That too can add to the existing overwhelm as energetically it can feel to mum (and especially to baby) that there is no *space* and too much *pressure*. By being aware of where I am placing my attention, I can choose whether to go in closer or perhaps move my attention further back. This could be just behind myself or even many miles away. When I find that ideal or 'sweetspot' it can be really supporting for the mother and baby. These initial steps, with practice, can take less than a minute.

I was now in a more relational space with Geraldine and Michael. At first, I was drawn to taking care of Geraldine. The initial step was to add cushions to her back, as she had been leaning forward to interact with her baby. With the support she relaxed and I then came back to baby.

Michael was crying in what felt like an inconsolable way: he had his eyes closed all the time. In the pre- and perinatal work when this happens, our understanding is that baby is accessing something in his own history: it may also be associated with something that is challenging in present time. The ability to be aware of time, and so differentiate our history from today, is not thought to be available to babies as their brains have not yet matured sufficiently. Thus, they are unable to perceive the difference between a past or present time. The result of not perceiving a future place means it is not possible to perceive that whatever is happening can change: for them it can feel that this place they are in is forever.

With Geraldine's permission, I let Michael know that I was going to pick him up. When we can in this work, we slow down in our interactions with babies and children to give them time to take in what we are saying – what is about to happen. Once I was holding Michael, I continued to orient myself to present time and use the Midspace exercise. I let him know that his mother was here and that we were moving to a different place. As I said this I was moving from one part of the room to another, where the lighting was different. In the different lighting, I said that the light had changed and he was now in a different place – that he was safe and that I was holding him. Within a few cycles, Michael stopped crying and opened his eyes and made good, clear eye contact with me. It was then just a matter of taking the few steps back to Geraldine. With Geraldine having physical support and Michael settled and in present time, it only took a short time for them to connect and settle into feeding.

Attunement, resonance and harmonic resonance

The term attunement has been part of psychological vocabulary for some time, as has resonance; Castellino uses the term harmonic resonance. I feel that each of the terms expresses how we humans can deeply connect with each other. However, as you will read, there are some differences between the terms in relation to what they cover.

Siegel (2010, p.34) writes about attunement mainly within the physiological aspects of brain and senses, particularly in what Porges calls the social engagement system. Having trained as an engineer, studied as a Polarity Therapist and read some research that is being conducted with energy fields within the human body, I hold an open curiosity towards how energy fields may also play a part in the attunement, resonance and harmonic resonance debate.

I feel that harmonic resonance provides the opportunity to incorporate both the psychological aspects of attunement and resonance with the energy fields as it is associated with the Polarity Therapy paradigm. Castellino has written about this in his text (Castellino 1996b). Harmonic resonance tends to combine attunement and resonance. For simplicity here in this and the next chapter, I will generally use attunement and resonance to describe this relationship between individuals unless quoting Castellino.

Siegel (2010, p.34) defines attunement as 'how we focus our attention on others and take their essence into our own inner world.' It is our ability to perceive another person's states while remaining aware of our own. So we not only have the ability to attune to ourselves but also to others.

Resonance adds another layer. Siegel (2010, pp.54–55) writes that resonance is when 'the observed takes in the observer having taken her in, and the two become joined'. Siegel continues that 'resonance moves us beyond understanding and into engagement'. I feel it is a relational dance.

Our ability to come into attunement and resonance with an infant or adult is perhaps one of the most important ways we have of being in relationship: of feeling connected to someone else. I consider it a significant resource. Castellino states:

> The key to support the family is to come into harmonic resonance and when the harmonic resonance is in the family the babies and children can thrive. (Castellino *et al.* 2013–2017)

Let us not forget the importance of clear boundaries in this work; otherwise we may end up merging with the other. Castellino (Castellino *et al.* 2013–2017) says: 'Harmonic resonance is when I can be separate from you yet feel you. If I am undifferentiated, I lose myself and become an empath.' We support families and small groups so that each participant can enter into attunement and resonance with a high degree of differentiation and what Castellino calls 'mutual support and cooperation' at the same time.

To enter into and maintain an attuned and resonant relationship requires that we have the capacity to remain responsive rather than reactive. As Siegel (2010, p.60) explains, when we are in reactive mode 'presence is shut down, attunement cannot happen, and resonance does not occur'. In other words, we need to develop a wider window of tolerance that supports our being responsive.

Attunement and resonance appear intimately connected with mirror neurons.[23] Van der Kolk (2014, p.58) writes that the discovery of mirror

---

23 Van der Kolk (2014, p.58) explains how a 'lucky accident' for a group of Italian researchers led to the discovery of mirror neurons. The researchers were monitoring the monkey's premotor area as part of their experiments. When the researcher was 'putting food pellets into a box', the 'monkey's brain cells were firing at the exact location where the motor command neurons were located'. This was at a time where the 'monkey wasn't eating or moving. He was watching the researcher, and his brain was vicariously mirroring the researcher's actions.'

neurons explains 'empathy, imitation, synchrony, and even the development of language'.

Being attuned with another is not just about being aware of another: it is much more comprehensive. According to Siegel (2010, p.34), it is about perceiving both the words and 'nonverbal patterns of energy and information flow', as well as 'seeing someone deeply, of taking in the essence of another person in that moment'. The outcome of this provides the parent or therapist with a *felt sense* of what the child or client is experiencing in the present moment. Or as Van der Kolk (2014, pp.111–112) puts it, 'it gives the baby the feeling of being met and understood'. It is this level of connection I believe that promotes a feeling of safety and security. This *understanding* that I am being seen: that I am not alone. I see our being able to come into attunement and resonance with another, especially in early life and in the development of a secure attachment, as a major source of resource and support in both the family and therapeutic settings.

Van der Kolk goes on to write about the sequence of delight, rupture, repair and new delight in an experiment by Ed Tronick.[24] The essence here was moving from an attuned relationship between mother and baby (delight) to where the baby pulled his mother's hair. This caused her to feel pain and anger, which disrupted the attuned relationship (i.e. rupture). His mother was able to swiftly shift from this state and together they re-established attunement (repair).

The loss of attunement here is caused by the difference between what the toddler expects as an outcome and what actually occurs. The effect of this is to cause a rapid change of state from the social connection into activation of the parasympathetic nervous system. Schore (2003, p.17) writes that this rapid transition from a positive to a negative state is represented by shame, and Siegel (2012, p.312) writes:

> Shame is thought to be based on the activation of the parasympathetic system (to an external 'No!') in the face of a highly charged sympathetic system (an internal 'Let's go!').

It is important to be aware that shame in terms of loss of attunement, of loss of expectation of being met with a smiling, joyous reflection from mum, is not the same as humiliation, where a child is shamed. Gerhardt (2015, p.67) makes the point that 'shame is an important dimension of socialization'.

---

24 A slightly different experiment, 'The Still Face' (Tronick 2009), also demonstrates the lack of attunement when the mother does not respond to her child.

She continues, 'what matters equally is the recovery from shame', which is in line with shifting from rupture to repair as I mentioned earlier. I believe there is something life-enhancing and resourcing in experiencing a rupture in a secure relationship; to have it be seen and then return to harmony. It creates the imprint or the 'knowing' that when things do go wrong or situations are uncomfortable, life can return to being an OK, attuned relationship.

The rapid recovery from shame and the loss of the regulatory relationship, while ideal, does not always happen. For some, the outcome can result in being left in rupture until they find a way out. This is a very different imprint. I have both seen and experienced forms of this with the pre- and perinatal work. On one occasion I was facilitating a group where I caused a rupture by 'getting something wrong'[25] for the client, and in so doing causing a disconnect in the attuned field. By pausing, clarifying what just happened, while providing space for the client's feelings where he can perceive he is being heard, the rupture was repaired and we returned to what I feel was a *strengthened* attuned relationship.

Being in attunement with another can also have a downside. Van der Kolk (2014, p.59) mentions how:

> …our mirror neurons also make us vulnerable to others' negativity so that we respond to their anger with fury or are dragged down by their depression.

For this reason, I suggest it is so important that we as therapists, and those who are part of the babies' and children's relationships, develop coherent narratives of our histories by making sense of our own ruptures and trauma imprints: moving from reaction to responsiveness; being clear of who I am and that I am separate from my client even in the attuned relationship.

To be attuned we have to be present. Castellino developed the Midspace exercise – a simple process we use for being present by orientating to the physical body. The process is used to support us and our clients to come into relationship with each part of our body and with ourselves in that moment.

We begin by allowing our awareness to be in our sacrum, through which we can connect to feeling the ground beneath us, supporting us. From there we orient to a place in our cranium that we can settle in. From within our cranium we can have awareness of the sky above and around us. We now have the connection between the support of the ground beneath us

---

25 In my experience, many times when I have initially thought that I had 'got it wrong' for a client, it has turned out to be a gift in supporting the resolution of part of his history.

up to our head: a central column from ground to head. It provides us with an awareness of our midline.[26]

Anna Chitty emphasizes the value of the term 'midspace' as an alternative to the more commonly used 'midline'. The signature of the midspace is stillness. For her, midspace incorporates midline but adds an important perceptual factor that supports access to deeper layers of the system.

Having established the midline or midspace, we now allow our attention to perceive and feel the left side of our body, then the midspace, then the right side. In the same way we then take our awareness to the back of our body, the midspace and then the front. Finally, we connect with a sense of our inside, midspace and outside. Castellino and Chitty refer to this process of moving to one place and then to the opposite side of the body as pendulation. We can go around this circuit as often as we feel we need to. As we pendulate between these different spaces in our body, we become more aware of the sensations and feelings held there; and as we deepen we can open to be with the underlying energies there. Our deepening in the midspace supports us to touch what Castellino calls the 'sweetspot'. The sweetspot opens us up to the possibility of accessing the Blueprint energy (see later in the chapter).

This is a useful exercise to support us and our clients to come back into being present: being in present time. With practice it takes just a short time to do it. Within the section on the core principles, Chapter 8, I describe how we develop the building blocks for attunement and harmonic resonance.

I would like to share with you a schematic representation of behavioural curves (Figure 7.8) that I came across earlier in my career. It is taken from Schore (1994, p.87), where he quotes Field (1985). The two curves in the figure show the differences between the attuned and misattuned infant–mother relationship. In the upper schematic (attuned), the mother provides stimulus to her child in relation to where his arousal level is. In this schematic, arousal is defined by the child's heart rate. To support him to remain within his window of tolerance she moves between providing stimulus and pauses (or lower levels of stimulus). The pace is such that her child can integrate the stimuli. It supports the modelling of her child's young nervous system.

---

26   The term 'midline' arose out of the cranial osteopathic and craniosacral field. It is first named during the development of the embryo, as the notochord develops. It 'acts as a place of orientation' (Kern 2001, p.106). Orientating to our midline is about orienting from our inside to the outside. It helps us to settle and it can also support those around us to be aware of their own midline.

The lower schematic shows the misattuned infant–mother relationship. Without attunement her child exceeds his window of tolerance and cries.

Whilst the text associated with the schematic refers to the infant–mother dyad, I suggest that it could be anyone in the primary caring relationship with the infant.

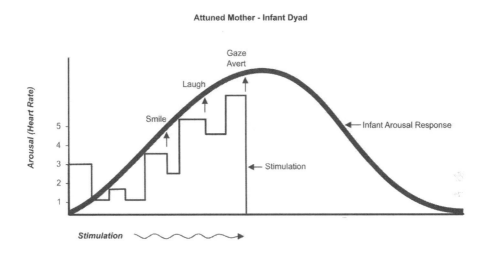

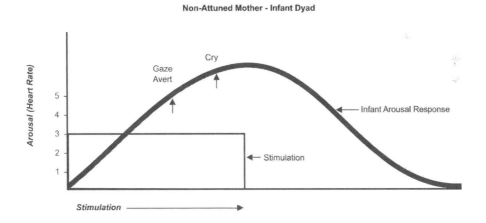

Figure 7.8 Schematic representation of behavioural curves

Gerhardt (2015, p.58) provides an additional layer to this attunement dance. She writes about the effect of the parent's nervous system on her baby:

> The baby's heart rate has been found to synchronise with the parent's heart rate; if she is relaxed and in a coherent state, so will the baby be.

Her autonomic nervous system in effect communicates with her baby's nervous system, soothing it through touch.

According to Gerhardt (2015, p.82), having emotional support in early life forms an important part in developing the nervous system and 'how stress is interpreted and responded to in the future'. Given that stress is now perceived to affect us in all aspects of our lives, there is an opportunity to make a huge difference by beginning with early care.

Relational tide

Our bodies have numerous rhythms that cycle continuously. In doing so, life and health are supported and maintained; examples of these rhythms are the heart beat and breathing. Less well known are the slow rhythms that osteopaths and the craniosacral therapy world have been paying attention to:

- Cranial rhythmic impulse (CRI)
- Mid-tide
- Long tide.

The CRI is the most rapid and superficial of these three rhythms; it moves between 8 and 12 cycles a minute and is involved with the structures of the body. In *gear shifting* down from CRI we arrive at the mid-tide. It is considered to be more energized than the CRI: it is said to contain the biodynamic potency of the system and has a frequency of about 2½ cycles per minute. A further step down takes us to what the old osteopaths called the long tide, and its frequency is about 100 seconds per cycle. These rhythms are discussed in Chapter 12.

As part of my interview with Castellino, he introduced his understanding of a further rhythm – a baseline rhythm that he calls the 'relational rhythm' (Castellino 2015b). He began to notice it as he paid attention to the pre- and perinatal imprints while working with families and small groups. He has measured it at about a 2½ minute cycle, although he has found that there can be some variation from person to person and group to group. He believes that it arises 'out of the energy that happens between people that are in relationship: especially babies, children and families'. He explained that 'this baseline rhythm has no charge on it. It is simple, it's neutral. It is happening because the whole universe is expanding and contracting.' 'It gives us access to the Blueprint energy.'

All these rhythms are illustrated in Figure 7.9.

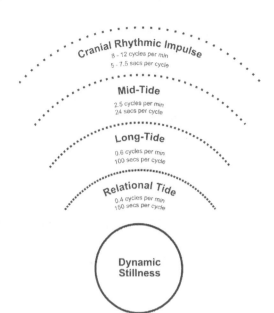

Figure 7.9 The Tides

Blueprint energy

The term Blueprint energy originates from the work of Dr Randolph Stone,[27] who developed Polarity Therapy. Polarity Therapy considers human life to be made up of both the physical anatomy as well as the *fine energy currents* of life. Stone writes:

> There are primal pattern energies and fields in our makeup, which are as true and essential to our function and life as a blueprint is to a well laid out structure or a mechanical design. (Stone 1985, p.104)

The Blueprint energy is considered by Castellino as a significant resource in working with the pre- and perinatal field. He describes it as the 'Polarity Principle in action'. It is present before we are conceived and is based on the expression of health. He described how 'It's the energy that helps and organises our consciousness. It organises the way our mind works. It organises the way our body shapes' (Castellino 2015b). It exists before all our other experiences are layered onto us in our life journey. These layers of experience might be a challenging pregnancy, birth, early life or ancestral patterns that

---

27   Stone was a contemporary of Dr William Sutherland, who developed cranial osteopathy from his perceptions and studies as an osteopath.

are expressed within our family surround. In these circumstances we might adapt and accommodate to the extent that we lose our connection with the Blueprint. We therefore may become more about the layers than who we truly are.

By reconnecting to this Blueprint energy, we reconnect with a time before the imprints that we have collected in this life. We are in relation to the health of our system and that supports us to integrate the trauma imprints as we pendulate between the trauma and the Blueprint.

Castellino (2015b) advises that 'if you attune to the Blueprint you will attune to the tides that are appropriate to the relationships'. In other words, when we are by ourselves we can access the Blueprint energy by being in the long tide. Within families or small-group settings we would be within the slower tide: the relational tide.

The need for the perception of feeling safe

Generally, when we feel safe, we are more able to be in loving relationship, and to be more present in our authentic self. When we do not feel this safety, or perceive it, we shift into survival and stress, as mentioned earlier in the section on the Polyvagal Theory. Our connection moves from loving relationship to a survival connection. In early life this is the difference between love and trauma bonding.

Porges (2013) notes that very young infants are less discriminatory with whom they interact with in respect of the social engagement aspect. That:

> …there is tremendous plasticity in the system for babies to be held by many different people. But as the baby gets older, the process of neuroception, which detects features of safety, becomes more and more selective in identifying familiarity and defining safety before the baby can be held.

Through different aspects such as the environment, social engagement, pacing, protection, clarity and overall holding of the therapeutic container, safety can begin to develop. Over time, with trust, developing the feeling of safety can grow and the infant or adult client and therapist can relax and be more open to the healing process.

In the next chapter we look at the Castellino-based approach to working with adults and families.

CHAPTER 8

SUPPORTING BABIES, CHILDREN AND THEIR FAMILIES ON THEIR JOURNEY OF INTEGRATION

David Haas

Approaches to working with babies, children and their families is a huge subject, so to keep some containment, this chapter focuses on some of the more important points. The essence of this work grew out of the need to create a space where babies and children could express themselves in relationship with their parents. Parents are also supported to develop coherent narratives for themselves as well as for their child. In other words, to differentiate what happened in the history from where they are right now. This beginning came in the form of Infant-centred Family Work and over time grew to add additional forms or structures of working. They are:

- Infant-centred Family Work (ICFW)

- Womb Surround Process Workshops (PWs)

- One-to-one sessions.

Creating a space, a *container*, for working with early life material, a time in our lives when we are vulnerable and our body systems are still developing, requires a particular structure. This container is provided by the core principles and the form. They developed out of the work of Infant-centred Family Work at the BEBA clinic in Santa Barbara, California, and Castellino's development of the Womb Surround Process Workshops. These are described in more depth later in the chapter. Castellino calls the core principles the 'rules of the game' and the form is the 'structure that allows practitioners and clients to be able to function and come into harmonic resonance'.

The PWs and one-to-one sessions are for adults. While this book is about working with babies and children, we must remember it is also important to work therapeutically with their parents and other primary carers.

The thread that links these different approaches is about integrating historic events that were overwhelming – traumatic. As previously discussed, whether an event is too much, and thus overwhelming/traumatic, is dependent on our resources. This in turn affects the width of the window of tolerance. There are two skills that are useful in supporting integration: pendulation and titration.

I mentioned pendulation in the previous chapter in the attunement, resonance and harmonic resonance section in relation to the exercise for establishing the resource of midspace. Peter Levine, as part of his writings on Somatic Experiencing®, explains it slightly differently:

> …the term 'pendulation' refers to a natural rhythm (of contraction and expansion) inherent within us that guides us back and forth between uncomfortable sensations, emotions, and images to more comfortable ones, allowing for new experiences and meanings to emerge… Pendulation is what keeps the momentum of change happening over time. (Levine and Kline 2007, p.93)

Titration, on the other hand, is about breaking up the stimulus into manageable pieces. In the previous chapter, in the section on attunement, resonance and harmonic resonance, I wrote about the attuned mother:

> …she moves between providing stimulus and pauses (or lower levels of stimulus). The pace is such that her child can integrate the stimuli.

She was able to interact with her baby so that he could remain within his window of tolerance. She managed that by titrating their interaction. In this way they maintain their relationship within the window of tolerance.

Infant-centred Family Work

It is clear that within one-to-one sessions there are only two people in the space: the therapist and the client. When a baby or a young child comes for a session, they always bring someone else with them. The therapist is now working with a group dynamic and so he needs to be aware and to be able to hold the different layers that can be present for each adult and infant. These layers may arise out of their relationship, and/or between them and the therapist. It can become confusing for the therapist, especially when working on their own, so having support in the session with a co-facilitator or assistant is a great benefit. While, as we have seen, the layers of support are really useful, it is a particular benefit when we are facilitating a session on our own: a layer of support may also be in the form of supervision following a session.

One of the challenges in supporting families to be in relationship is that in our society today there is so much information about how to be during pregnancy: how to birth, how to parent your child, and so on. The information just keeps on coming. However, it is very much *outside-in* information. There is a tendency for it to engage the mind and so parents can lose connection with their *felt sense*[1] – their body knowing – and as such it can be confusing and overwhelming. Within the pre- and perinatal work, we support the parents and their children to slow down and connect with their own *knowing* first: with their impulse. This impulse is the *inside-out* information and it is their *body knowing*. For this reason, we wait to see what unfolds during therapy, rather than be prescriptive about what should happen.

Castellino acknowledges embryologist Jaap Van de Wal in his perception that the mother's body during pregnancy is the outer layer of the baby; in other words, the baby's outer body is perceived as the mother. In our work, we feel that the newborn infants and prenates in the womb are undifferentiated beings:

> They are not saying this is mum and this is me. They experience all of that as a developing self. The prenate in the womb is having the experience of the mother. (Castellino 2015b)

Within Infant-centred Family Work, the attention for the turn is with the infant. We look to support her to share her story and feelings in relationship

---

1   Bodily *felt sense* is a term that arose out Eugene Gendlin's therapeutic focusing work. Gerhardt (2015, p.73) quotes Gendlin, 'who describes how "words that flow out of a feeling" are the kind that make you say *"that's what it's all about!"'*. Being able to connect and listen to the *felt sense* and then express it in words provides the linkage between the left and right brain. It provides a coherent narrative in relation to the feeling, and as Gerhardt goes on to say, 'The mind is no longer trapped in unregulated emotional arousal, but is able to use all its resources, particularly those of the left brain, to regulate feelings.'

with her parents. As part of this, we support the parents to differentiate their needs from their prenate, baby and children. Castellino shares an example of differentiation of a pregnant mother who is having a hard day. The differentiation statement might be: 'I am having a hard day and it's not you. You are not causing this.' If on the other hand the mother does not make this differentiation statement, then the baby may have the imprint that he/she caused it. Where the mother does make the differentiation statement then the baby can get an imprint of the differentiation. Castellino goes on to say:

> What we see is that children who come from mothers who do that, those children start to differentiate the difference between themselves and their parent's ways sooner than you and I did. (2015b)

Form for working with families

The form for working with families differs from that of adults. With families, the parents hold a unique position. They are the main attachment figures for the infant. We take case histories, not only for the child, but also for each of the parents. Each parent names what their intention is for their child: they may be different. The parents' intention sets the container for the session. If we stopped at this point there is the possibility that too much attention is placed on the child to achieve an outcome. So we also ask the parents, what do you want for yourselves? In so doing, it places attention on themselves, which in turn supports their child to relax.

The therapist meets initially with the parents to go through the case histories and provide any clarifications needed. We also go through the core principles. It is an initial place of meeting and beginning the journey in deepening the therapeutic relationship. We are building the container and layers of support.

The next session is with the infant and the parents. We look to support the infant to share her story and feelings in relationship with her parents. We have found that babies and children organize themselves in relation to how their parents are doing. Remember that the parents are usually the main attachment figures in their child's life. In the infant's perception, her parents are her way of thriving in this world. Amongst other things, they provide food, nurture and safety. Where the parents are not coping well, such as difficulty relating with one another, in an anxious space, or mum suffering with postpartum depression, infants will attempt to compensate in the relationship. They need to stay attuned to get their needs met. Babies and children can compensate. This might be manifested as them being really good or behaving in other ways that reduce the demand on their parents. Some of the ways they may try to achieve this are by:

- trying to be ahead of their years

- holding back and internalizing their feelings

- being really good

- sleeping more than expected.

In this kind of situation, it becomes difficult for them to show their story as their belief is that it might become too much for their parents and thus threaten their ability to thrive. The more the parents get supported to relax, and are available for attunement and harmonic resonance, the easier it becomes for the infant to show what they need. In sessions we see that as this support happens for the parents, their child is more able to open up.

BEBA (2016) describes the essence of the session work as follows:

> In BEBA, infants and children replay the initial traumatic event over and over until they master it. Adults in Process Workshops likewise physically recreate early events but at a slower pace and are well resourced with support from others. The replay is done with the body, not just with the neocortical mind. The goal is to affect the amygdala directly. Words are used to describe what is happening physically to link the amygdala and the neocortex. 'You are moving through the stuck place.' Once the initial trauma has been resolved, 'cues' no longer stimulate a fight or flight reaction. The infant/ child/adult not only is not afraid of the 'cue', he or she enjoys the process of mastery and seeks ever-increasing challenges.

It is within the session that we bring together the resources, such as the long tide, relational tide, Blueprint and attunement/harmonic resonance, to support developing the coherent narratives as the trauma imprints move to integration.

The following lists are a sample from BEBA (2016). They indicate some of the different aspects: causes, signs and parental response. A copy of the complete list can be viewed in Appendix A. A partial list of indications of non-traumatized and traumatized neonates is provided later in this chapter and a fuller list in Appendix B.

- Some of the known causes of early trauma include:
    - » Maternal stress, fear or depression during pregnancy or after birth
    - » Child not wanted for some or part of the pregnancy
    - » NICU experience with all accompanying medical interventions
    - » Near-death experience or deprivation of oxygen.
- Some of the signs older children exhibit after experiencing trauma include:
    - » Hyperactivity
    - » Coordination and balance problems
    - » Speech delays
    - » Nightmares
    - » Health challenges such as asthma and seizures.
- Common parental responses to a child's early trauma might be:
    - » Overwhelm
    - » Shame/guilt
    - » Anxiety
    - » Helplessness
    - » Conflict between parents
    - » Difficulty asking for support.

As the sessions progress, the parents' early trauma history imprints may arise. These are not explored in the session unless they are relevant to the child's story. The parents will have sessions either by themselves or as a couple.

Whilst the infant-centred work was developed for infants, I have also used it in working with families with teenagers. Teenagers sit in the place between being a child and an adult. For them there can be the desire to be the adult and then getting into situations where it is too much for them. They need to have a stable and safe place that they can go to as a reference. Ideally this is their parents or other responsible adults. Neufeld and Maté (2006, p.7) wrote how young people were turning away from mothers, fathers and other responsible adults for guidance, modelling and instruction. They were turning to their peers for this support, and Neufeld and Maté coined the phrase *peer orientation*. In our support of parents to integrate their histories and come into attuned relationship with each other, I suggest they become more available to their children. I believe that where there is an attuned, safe space available, there is more opportunity for the teenager to reorient to their parents and away from peer orientation.

Womb Surround Process Workshops and Individual Sessions

The work with adults developed out of the Infant-centred Family Work, so the same level of holding to support very open and vulnerable newborns and infants is maintained.

Process workshops are small-group settings with typically no more than seven participants, held over several days to explore early imprinting that is affecting present-day life. The initial phase of the workshop develops the structure and, as Castellino puts it, 'with the intention of creating a safe and nurturing "womb surround"'. Each participant has the opportunity to have a turn where he can explore emotional and physical patterns from early life. As a turn develops, so layers of the surround, made up of some or all of the participants, develop to support the turn person's process. The slow tempo provides the space, together with the contact and support, for the turn person to develop a coherent narrative of his early imprints and in so doing move towards healing. More information on the form for the process workshop is described after the core principles later in this chapter.

Individual sessions are available for those who prefer to work on their own with their therapist. The form for these sessions is a reduced version of that used within process workshops.

We will now look at the core principles and the form that are the structures of the session. While there are the three forms of therapy containers mentioned above, the core principles remain the same and the form of the session changes. The two structures are shown separately, and it is their interweaving that provides the environment, the *space*, that supports each person present.

The core principles

When Ray Castellino and Wendy McCarty created BEBA, they developed a set of core principles, also referred to as core values by other colleagues, to create a safe container for all those present. These core principles were included as part of Castellino's development of the Womb Surround Process Workshops (PWs) and have been added to over the years. Castellino calls the principles the 'rules of the game' and the form is the 'structure that allows practitioners and clients to be able to function and come into Harmonic Resonance [HR]'. He further defines HR in relationship as 'when I can be separate from you and yet feel you' (Castellino *et al.* 2013–2017).

Critical to this pre- and perinatal work is for each person, infant or adult, to feel safe. That is not just a cognitive understanding but a somatic – of the body – *felt sense*. That might feel like an open and flowing space in our body or perhaps a settling. When we feel safe our survival behaviours are not activated, we are within our functional range – our window of tolerance – and we sit within the social engagement system; within this space we are able to be responsive rather than reactive. As we move out of our survival mechanism, so the level of the stress hormone cortisol reduces. This provides space to support relationship and increases the hormone oxytocin.

The core principles are always shared either prior to, or at the beginning of, the first session. Within the family work they are shared initially with the parents and then are brought in to the sessions with infants and children as appropriate: usually, rather than explaining as we would for adults, the facilitators model the core principles for the children during the sessions. An example of this is under the principle of choice below: here, in Martin's session, I model holding the boundary that he initially wants to push through. As you will see in the descriptions that follow, each core principle has an underlying reason for being included.

Principle of mutual support and cooperation

> Mutual support is the ability to be supportive of one's self and of others at the same time. When groups of people including families live in this principle children grow into strong autonomous adults. (Castellino 2015c)

Castellino has more recently refined this statement to include, 'The support is mutual, it is cooperative and not at the expense of the self'.

I believe that to develop relationship requires cooperation: a willingness to move from our usual position. Feeling safe and supported increases our ability to move more into health. To be cooperative we need to be able to *let down and settle in our self.* Mutual support and cooperation evolves from the felt sense within our body. We can stand in our position and not move from our beliefs and perceptions, but from this place there is little or no room for change. Combining mutual support with cooperation supports us to be there for ourselves and for others; to be more vulnerable and more likely to be responsive in the relationship rather than reactive.

Castellino explains that: 'It is in the Blueprint energy we will find our commonality. If we find our commonality we find a new way into mutual support and cooperation.' Castellino *et al.* (2013–2017, p.3)

Käppeli shared a case with me that demonstrates mutual support and cooperation in action: parents-to-be were preparing for the birth of their baby and they came for a session. The father, Thomas, said that he did not feel he would be able to be present at the birth because he reacts strongly to blood. Käppeli suggested that first he speaks to his unborn baby and lets her know that he very deeply wants to be at her birth for her and also to support her mother: that he also explains that because of his fear of blood he may not be able to stay and be present in the room. In this way he is letting his baby know so that she can orient to her father's position. In the event that Thomas feels he has to leave, then his baby can have an understanding that she did not cause it. It brings a clarity to the field. Käppeli also suggested to Thomas that he asks a friend to sit outside the delivery room with him and in doing so provide another layer of support. After the birth, Thomas shared with Käppeli that in the end he was able to stay and be present for the whole birth, even though there was a lot of blood. So Thomas was able to take care of himself (with external support) and be supportive of both his partner and their baby.

Principle of choice

When I am facilitating a session, I may have an idea – a suggestion – for the client. An example would be my wanting to physically move closer. As part of the principle of choice, I ask the client to take a moment and see how it feels. If he doesn't feel it is wholly right then I encourage and support him to say 'no'. A similar situation could arise with any participant in the session requesting, for example, some form of support from someone else.

It seems simple. A 'yes' or a 'no'. But how many of us find saying 'no' a challenge? It is usually easier to say 'yes', even though it brings its own challenges. When we mean 'no' and say 'yes' it creates a split between our mind and our somatic body, resulting in tension: it is a stress and creates confusion within us and for those around us. Why say 'yes' when we really mean 'no'?

I suggest there are number of reasons. Fear of not being liked or loved; that the other person may leave; the emotional upset we believe may result; or fear of being shamed are some examples and there are probably more.

A 'no' that comes from within us – from our felt sense – sets a boundary. This 'no' creates safety and is more supportive of the relationship than when we have an *inside* 'no' and say an *outside* 'yes'. With a 'no' that is clear and grounded within an individual, the person is telling me that this is as far as he is prepared to go – this is as close as he is willing to have me come. When this is acknowledged and kept to, we feel safer; we are more likely to trust the other person.

In working with traumatic imprints it is important that the client is able to sit on the edge of his material. In everyday life the trauma imprint can just take us back into the trauma memory and we get lost in it for a while. By sitting on the edge of the trauma we have the opportunity to dissipate the shock energy of the trauma and begin to integrate and heal. How close we are willing to approach this edge depends on our trust of the therapist, our feeling safe, and in part this comes from our 'no', pause, or our 'stop', being heard and followed. It's like being invited to go to the edge of a cliff with the therapist. If I know he will stop immediately I say so, I am more likely to go closer to the edge. If I don't have that trust, I will wait further from the edge.

Boundaries are important because without them we cannot have relationship. To have relationship we need to have a sense of our self that is separate from another. When there is no separation then we are one;

the same; merged. With clear boundaries and feelings of safety, we have the opportunity to deepen our relationship into intimacy. Boundaries also help us to orient in space and time, to know where we are. This can aid us to differentiate our history from the present moment.

Babies and children need clear boundaries where they are met. With clear boundaries we create safe containers for them to play and investigate in. Having a safe container, babies and children have the opportunity to let go of their fear and freely explore their potential. As the child grows, so does the container. This same philosophy is useful in the workplace. Boundaries need to be inherently flexible. Some boundaries can have greater flexibility whereas others need to be more firm. This relates to mutual support and cooperation, discussed earlier. Rigid/trauma boundaries cause us to 'bounce off' them. In my practice I have noticed a particular sequence of events that can occur in relation to boundaries and children.

This is a typical example. Martin was about two years old when he came with his mother for a session. They entered the therapy space and I closed the door. Martin spent some minutes exploring the room space and then he returned to the closed door with the intention to explore the other spaces in the building.

As I held the door closed, he pulled at the handle and began to lightly kick at the door. I acknowledged what he wanted and his feelings and said that for now the door is closed and he will be able to go out later. He went away and then returned. This time he also tried to encourage his mother's help and she reinforced holding the boundary. We went through the same cycle. He did this once more and then left the door, joined his mother and began to show us a deep part of his history.

Babies and children show their preferences and choices: it is always important to at least acknowledge what they are wanting even if it is sometimes necessary to say 'no'. I suggest that being met with a clear, strong boundary that was held whilst remaining in relationship with Martin – acknowledging what he wanted and his feelings – created a sense of safety, of protection. It is important for every child to have a felt sense of being protected. This felt sense can deepen and grow over time with similar experiences. It can be recalled when needed to support self-regulation. If as children we experience what it feels like to have clear, coherent boundaries held for us, then as we become older I believe we are more able to accept boundaries in a responsively conscious way rather than reactively.

Principle of brief frequent eye contact

I have found in the Womb Surround Process Workshops that I facilitate for adults how easy it is for the group's attention to focus intently on the person taking a turn. This can happen for a variety of reasons. The effect of this level of attention can feel overwhelming for the person who is taking the turn. One of the tools we use to shift this attention is what is termed brief frequent eye contact (BFEC).

BFEC developed as part of the BEBA clinic skill set where it was perceived that parents were losing relational connection with each other as their attention was fully on their child. That degree of attention may also be too much for their child and affect his ability to remain within the social engagement system. We suggest to parents that they make eye contact with each other for some moments from within the place of mutual support and cooperation about every two and a half minutes. We have found that this aids the couple in developing a connected and supportive relationship with each other, as well as reducing the level of attention on their child. This in turn supports their child to remain within, or return to, the social engagement system. This two-and-a-half-minute cycle is called the long tide in craniosacral therapy and is a deeply settling resource.

As part of making BFEC, we may also use the Midspace exercise. In doing so it helps us to be more present and grounded in our body and more responsive rather than reactive to those around us. Together with some physical contact such as holding hands, the parents become attuned with each other and from this place return to relationship with their child.

Within a process workshop there is only one person taking a turn. The remaining participants form energetically what we call the *surround*. As they use BFEC between each other, they strengthen the energy in the surround, which is a metaphor for the uterus itself.

Principle of making contact: touch with attention

Touch is one way we come into relationship with another. Our experience of touch in our early lives was not necessarily always resourcing. It may have happened too fast for us or when we weren't wanting it. Perhaps we even felt it was painful. Within the core principles we seek to make contact in a resourcing and supportive way that also pays attention to the recipient's choice to receive or not receive contact. We are empowering the recipient in their choice.

When I am facilitating in a process workshop and have the impulse that I would like to provide some physical support to the turn person, I first direct my attention to the turn person and make eye contact with her. Then I let her know that I would like to make contact and where this might be; it may be a foot, or their lower back or hand. She then has the opportunity to negotiate my offer and either to accept it or to say 'no'. If she is happy to have the contact, then I will slowly move to where I can make the contact. I will let her know as I am about to make contact. When the time comes to remove the contact, I will let her know before I take my hand away. On a subtle level it means there is less likelihood of it being a shock.

This level of connection can be very useful in supporting some re-patterning of early experiences. However, there are also times when this level of connection is not necessary or perhaps appropriate. For example, if the participant has requested contact, or contact needs to be made quickly to support or keep him safe.

Within the Infant-centred Family Work, I tend to slow down in myself to meet the babies and children at their pace. The approach of getting permission with children where they are able to voice their response is the same as has been described with adults. Where they are not able to, or if I am working with babies, I rely on my being in attunement/harmonic resonance with them, in order to get a felt sense of their response. I then name it, and watch how they respond. I have noticed how some babies turn their head or body away, or perhaps withdraw their foot. At that point I pause and acknowledge what they did and I make it clear that I understand that is a 'no'. After a few moments they look back at me and I check in again. If I get the same response, then I will stop. Other times they remain with good, clear eye contact and I let them know I will make contact. For me, I feel that once they get that they are being *seen* and *heard*, they are more willing for me to come closer to what might be a sensitive place for them.

Having touch and physical contact has been found to have additional relational benefits through the release of oxytocin. According to Kerstin Moberg:

Touch and physical contact initiate a reinforcing cycle and produce increased secretion of oxytocin; this makes us more curious and interested in establishing contact, and, this in its turn, releases still more oxytocin, and so on. (Moberg 2011, p.124)

To summarize, the important steps in making contact are:

- Directing the attention

- Stating the impulse

- Negotiating

- Acting

- Integrating.

The steps are the same whether we go in or out of contact.

Principle of self-regulation: the pause

The primary purpose of the pause principle is to support self-regulation. When we are able to self-regulate, we operate within our natural functional range – the window of tolerance. In this place we can integrate experiences in the moment as we live it. Above all, it supports us to remain in relationship and be more present in ourselves. It is difficult for parents to be in relationship and hold an attuned space for their child when they are in reaction with themselves or each other.

What happens without the pause? Remember that traumatic imprints arise out of our inability to digest and integrate events in our life. Within the imprint are the *locked-in* feelings, sensations and shock energy from the event. When trauma occurs, our naturally integrated yet differentiated brain loses its interconnectedness. So the different sections of the brain continue to function but they don't communicate with each other in the same way. There is a change in the level of relationship; feelings and sensations remain but there is no autobiographical memory. There is no coherent narrative for the feelings and sensations to be oriented to. Each time our unconscious activates the feelings and sensations in response to a perceived fear state, there is nothing to tell us that it is from our history and we therefore feel it is to do with present time. To those around us, and maybe for ourselves too, we don't understand why we are reacting by becoming angry, tearful or shifting to physical or dissociated flight. We are acting out of context of the current situation. We are instead *acting out* from an earlier time in our history.

Within the realm of the trauma imprint our behaviour is that of survival. This is a constricted, and probably a *speed up*, place as we focus in on the challenge. In order to move back into our window of tolerance and to have our left and right brain come back into relationship so we can integrate our experience, we need to create space and to slow down. We need to slow down to the pace of our younger, challenged self. Or maybe we need to slow down to support the child that is with us when we are rushing to get out of the door. Going at the child's pace reduces the chances of her being overwhelmed and becoming reactive. The pause creates space so we can slow down and can also remove the trigger of our activation. Castellino advises that:

> If we are able to go at the speed of the slowest part, then we will have the whole experience. (Castellino *et al.* 2013–2017)

He goes on to explain about when the pause is not available:

> If I have no way to regulate the tempo my nervous system will compress and jam. That compromises my ability to self-regulate. My system will either shut down or over-stimulate and go to fight–flight.

When we call a pause in a session, the agreement is that everyone stops what they are doing. In this way, whatever actions that were touching our earlier history are removed and our nervous system returns to its natural window of tolerance. We settle and are more able to be in present time and respond rather than react. We move out of stress and survival and back into relationship. At this point we release the pause and we carry on from where we were prior to the pause being called.

It can sometimes feel difficult to call a pause. We might feel we need to keep up with the others, or that it feels uncomfortable in some way to interrupt what is going on. Sometimes during a workshop, participants don't want to call a pause in case it interrupts the turn person's journey. However, the opposite can be true. If a participant is willing to call a pause for himself, then we pause, see what is needed and then continue. The participant taking care of himself by calling a pause may well be supporting the turn person getting something they did not have in their early life: perhaps somebody in their early life that was unable, say, to pause and self-regulate. The great thing about working with history is that calling a pause is like hitting the pause button on a video. Once the pause is lifted, the story just continues with no lost information.

It is important to remember that the pause is not about controlling the other person, it is about taking care of myself so that I can integrate some of my historic shock energy, begin to differentiate my historic trauma imprint material from present time, and above all stay present and remain in relationship. Babies and children can show us their need for a pause in various ways, perhaps turning their head away, or a child choosing to take herself to a different space in the room where it is quieter. As adults we can name it for them and pause with them.

I have worked with babies and toddlers who have suffered with convulsions and other challenges. By sitting and holding them within a pause, within the long tide, while naming each part of the convulsion cycle, we found that the convulsions reduced. In families, parents need to claim a pause when:

- they feel overwhelmed

- something does not feel safe

- the communication is confusing or lost.

Principle of self-care

Taking care of ourselves is of primary importance. It is part of self-regulating. Some basic functions of self-care are having enough to eat and being hydrated, feeling safe enough to sleep or rest, go to the toilet, and that our environment feels OK. Self-care is a foundation of the five-layered Hierarchy of Needs as developed by Maslow (1954). In our early life we depend on others to support us with care. We let them know when we are hungry or thirsty, are fearful, and so on. Our carers support us to self-regulate and settle in ourselves. When we don't get our self-care needs met, we move into more stress and reactivity. As I mentioned in the previous chapter, Castellino established that ideally we need two layers of support to settle: to let down and deepen. A mother is there to support her baby, her partner supports her, and so on.

Self-care is also about being able to accept support, although not everyone is open to receiving or able to ask for support. For some, early experiences in life of being expected to do it on their own, or a belief that 'I might be too much', can lead to a need to do it on their own. However, to try and do everything on our own can be stressful and challenge our ability to be present in relationship.

Principle of confidentiality

Confidentiality supports us to be vulnerable and to share places in ourselves that we would normally stay away from. With an agreement of confidentiality, we can feel more in control of how our story is shared. If a participant of a Womb Surround Process Workshop wishes to talk about their session outside the group, they are free to do so. However, if they want to speak about someone else's session, then they need to ask their permission first. I usually suggest that the person being asked takes a moment before responding with a 'yes' or 'no', and if they are happy to have the material shared then be clear what is being shared and to whom. Once it is out of the box it is difficult to put it back inside!

This level of confidentiality is also held within individual and family sessions. It is also important that confidentiality is held within families outside the sessions. As an example, we have noticed that where a mother is holding her baby and discusses the birth with someone else, the baby may become activated and express his feelings, even if he was asleep. Mum's labour and baby's birth are intimate processes between them. Sharing the story with others needs permission from mother and an awareness of what is OK for baby.

Principle of being welcomed

This additional core principle was included by Käppeli. This is about being welcomed, seen and heard; that you are welcome with your feelings and with your thoughts just as you are. This is about being met and accepted for who we are, and as such I feel it promotes a layer of settling. Initially we need to find and then go to the place in ourselves where we really feel that we can welcome from. Then we can share it. Käppeli names the core principle of being welcomed first. He considers that this core principle, together with mutual support and cooperation, forms the container for the remaining core principles.

The form of a session

As mentioned before, depending on the type of therapy session, ICFW, PW or individual sessions, the form will differ. The example provided here is based on the PW form. Aspects of the form, such as intention, have been touched on within the earlier description of an ICFW session. While Castellino calls this structure 'The Form', Käppeli and Regina Bücher[2] refer to it as the *gestalt*[3] of the session: they describe it as having an aliveness – an energy flow. Gestalt, they say, is about having an intention that is the beginning and then going through the process to an end place where the intention, or part of the intention, is complete; one feels somatically that the intention is complete.

Within the PPN work, it is easy to lose oneself in the sea of process. The structure of the form supports the client, the surround and the practitioner to reorient to present time. In doing so it provides the opportunity to differentiate the history from today. Each layer of the form builds on the previous layers, developing the container safety. In what follows here within this chapter, I provide some basic information about the form in order to provide some understanding of the concepts: more comprehensive information is provided within other documents and writings that fall outside the scope of this book.

Check-ins

Check-ins provide a point of reference in the session or process workshop. A check-in tells where you are in your life today; in this moment. It is for you to share how you are right now. Is there something going on for you that you want to name? Perhaps there is some activation? It is also a place to make a statement as to what kind of support would help you for the session. This is particularly useful for family and group work as everyone gets to know what you need: hearing what is going on for you provides the opportunity for everyone else to be able to differentiate your material from theirs. It helps to reduce tension and for each person to be seen as much as they choose.

2   Regina Bücher is a pre- and perinatal therapist and pedagogue for children with special needs in Germany.
3   Colman (2015) states that gestalt is: 'A perceptual configuration or structure that possesses qualities transcending the sum of its constituent elements or parts and that cannot be described simply in terms of its parts.' Put more simply by Tudor, Merry and Dryden (2002), it is: 'An organized whole that is perceived as more than the sum of its parts.'

Parents have fed back to me how useful even a brief check-in has been for them in their relationship. Just taking some moments at different times of their day has enhanced their ability to remain in relationship and then together to be present for their children.

The first session, or the beginning of the process workshop, tends to cover all the points. In follow-up sessions, or for process workshops at the beginning of each day, they tend to be an essence statement such as: 'I'm sleeping well and have had a good few days.' There is also space for clients to share more if they need: particularly if they are feeling activated. When check-ins are missed, it can lead to the group or family not understanding why members are behaving in the way they are. When we are able to understand their behaviour, I believe there is greater opportunity to be present with support and loving compassion rather than reaction.

The check-in can be important for people to orient to the present and to what we are going to do just now, for example having a session. The check-in does not belong to the form itself but it is a supportive element of the whole process.

The form structure

To give you an awareness of the form structure I have listed each of the nine aspects and will look at a couple in some more depth:

- Willingness to start a session

- Discovery of whose turn it is

- Affirmation of one's turn

- Intention for the session

- Relevant history

- Main body of session (action phase)

- Integration phase

- Group sharing

- Debriefing of the session.

Every group or family will move through the form in their own unique way. How much time is taken on each part will be dependent on the stories – the narratives, that are conscious or unconscious – that each person brings; how both individually and in combination they have an effect. Each part is important, as is the order. Different parts of the form may in themselves resonate with early times in the participants' history, such as the discovery of whose turn it is. Participants are not chosen to take a turn. The space is held for the discovery to come from the individuals' impulse and their own choice.

I have always been fascinated how each part of the form can have a correlation, a resonance, to sequences of preconception, gestation, birth and so on. The turn discovery is no exception. Käppeli considers the turn discovery as connected, resonating to the preconception period. He feels that 'the soul energy' knows the right time to come into life. Where the parents are not clear that it is the right time, then in the turn discovery setting, it can take longer for a participant in the group to know that it is his or her turn. So the process for discovering whose turn it is can either be a short process or it can expand to fill the whole turn.

As mentioned in the Infant-centred Family Work, the intention creates the container to work in; it provides direction. Within the main body of the session, we transition into the more active phase of the session. The client's story can unfold in a variety of ways based on the intention. Throughout this phase the integration of the trauma imprints continues. This occurs by titrating the imprint and by pendulating between the states of resource and overwhelm.

Castellino (2015c, p.38) lists a number of activities that may be worked on within this part of the turn:

- Womb surround

- Subtle movement showing implicit somatic memory

- Prenatal, conception or gestation exploration

- Exploration of a dream

- Somatic birth process

- Post-birth supported attachment

- Other trauma work

- Ancestral history

- CPBT (Castellino Prenatal and Birth Training) family constellation exploration

- Dynamic creative opposition.

Dynamic creative opposition (DCO) was developed by Castellino and is a way of coming into relationship. In the process of translating it into German, Käppeli and Bücher came up with the descriptive term *vitalizing resistance*. It is about being met with a level of physical contact that is neither overpowering nor underwhelming. It is, as in Goldilocks and the three bears, *just right*! In order to access certain somatic material, we need to create some physical resistance. In this case it is not fixed and rigid, rather flexible, responsive and dynamic. This resistance is a boundary and supports the client to sit on the edge of his material and titrate it in a resourced way. It supports the client to orientate, to know where they are, and to build the belief from the inside that 'I can manage it'. An example of where DCO can be used would be in accessing the birth process. DCO can range from very strong resistance and contact with the full body to subtle delicacy of touch between the little fingers. DCO also is useful in working with children who have experienced interventions during pregnancy and birth such as Caesarean sections or anaesthesia.

There will come a point within the session where a natural settling arises where either the full intention, or part of it, has been met. At this point we check in with the client where he feels he is with his intention.

I have written about the importance of developing the coherent narrative in relation to our imprints. As part of the form, we conclude with a debrief of the session. It is a time to develop integration between the left and right hemispheres of the brain and so to integrate the feelings and sensations with cognitive understanding.

CASE STUDY: INTENTIONS, BOUNDARIES AND BEING SEEN

I would like to share a case history about a client, Jeremiah (not his real name), which demonstrates the importance of boundaries with respect to setting intentions.

Jeremiah had been seeing me for some time and had always been seemingly comfortable in naming intentions for his sessions. We reached a point where he found it difficult to have an intention and became very reactive at even the mention of the word. In following the principle of choice, I acknowledged his 'no' and supported him to share just as he wanted. Initially, I was not concerned about this, as it is possible that even just finding an intention is actually the intention for the session. As this not wanting to have an intention carried on for some time, I became curious as to what was underpinning it.

In his early life and into his teenage years, Jeremiah had experienced a lack of boundaries from his parents. His parents' own patterns were such that they were unable to differentiate their material from his: boundaries were fuzzy or non-existent. He felt that that there was no space to have intentions for himself that were different from his parents.

During our work together I continued to hold clear boundaries for him, acknowledged what he wanted and differentiated my feelings and sensations from his. As time progressed, he began to develop a sense of his adult self in present time that was separate from his younger self. It was at this time that he began to access his feelings of anger from his younger self around having an intention. Jeremiah later shared how he had felt around intention sharing:

> 'An intention was expected, so I needed to come up with one to justify why I was coming for therapy. That was the framework. My younger self did his piece of being compliant! And over time, my younger self felt safe enough to express the anger of having to fit into someone else's framework for attention.'

He went on to say in relation to boundaries:

> 'As I began to experience what it was like to safely be seen and appreciated as a separate being with separate needs, wants and intentions, I developed an increasing sense of self.'

And his underpinning belief was:

> 'There was always this deep-seated belief that I am fundamentally, terribly bad or wrong.[4] Not having the reflection of seeing joy in another's eye in my childhood made it hard/impossible to rejoice in my own existence, feeling like my core is rotten. Having an intention would have meant being seen. Being truly seen would be awful as the belief is that they would see how awful I am.
>
> 'So best not to have a clear intention, best not to be seen, best not to exist.'

---

4   Jeremiah had shared earlier in therapy how his parents had not been married when they became pregnant. They then had to marry and his father had blamed his mother for getting it wrong and not preventing the pregnancy. Jeremiah felt that in the undifferentiated family space it formed part of the reason for his feeling that he 'had done something terribly wrong'.

As the therapy continued and the therapeutic relationship deepened, we reached a place where Jeremiah could perceive a look from me that in his words:

> '…felt to me as if you were proud of something that I did. A look of wonderment and joy and pride. To be looked at like that, to have that reflection – I felt worthy of existing.'

With this shift came another step in his ability to relate in a way that was more in line with the secure attachment style. As he developed in his inner felt sense of being worthy and with a clearer sense of boundaries, Jeremiah began to feel safe enough to allow himself to be seen. In this way he felt more comfortable to have an intention and to name it in relationship with someone else.

Personal work and supervision

As therapists, our ability to be able to sit with a client in the pre- and perinatal field requires us to work with our own history and trauma imprints, particularly those from our own early life journey. In this way we are less likely to be activated and reactive with our clients as they show us their history in their journey to heal.

In providing a layer of support to our clients, it is necessary that we too feel the benefits of support. With support we get to let down and deepen with our clients. Support can come in different ways. For the therapist, particularly when working in the PPN field, I feel that supervision is a necessary layer of support. In my early days as a bodyworker I did not have supervision in place. I have shared below the outcome.

I had been working as a craniosacral therapist at a time when working with babies was relatively new. I was only aware of one or two practitioners in this specialized field at that time. Also, as a bodyworker (I was also a polarity therapist), I did not really understand the need for supervision at that time. I thought that was something that psychotherapists and counsellors needed to do, as they dealt with psychological issues concerning things such as transference and counter-transference (transference being where the client has past emotional content reactivated, and transfers it onto the therapist). For example, in the client/therapist environment, the transference of the client's anger to his mother when he was a child is transferred to his therapist today. Counter-transference is the therapist's response from her past emotional content that is reactivated in relation to the client's transference.

I had been working with a mother and her baby and the previous sessions had been progressing well. I went on a further course for working with babies and on my return began to put my new learning into practice. From the moment I began working differently with this baby, she began to cry. It seemed that whatever I did made no difference. I felt terrible. What had I done? My work was about supporting healing with love and helping my clients move towards health and away from the pain. I felt inadequate; I could do nothing it seemed to make it better. I questioned my ability as a therapist.

After the session I took myself off for supervision and with support began to make sense of not only my own trauma imprints from my early life but also the effect they were having on my therapeutic relationship with my client. As I became more able to differentiate these historic patterns from today, it became easier for me to remain settled and be present for my clients: to be responsive rather than reactive in supporting them to integrate their trauma imprints.

CASE STUDY: FAMILY SESSION

I have spoken about different aspects of this work and I would now like to share with you how this unfolds with a family I have been treating. This section has come from an interview I had with the parents. To protect family confidentiality, names and certain other information have been changed. I am grateful to them for their permission to include this part of their story.

The family consists of mum Joanna, dad Jonathan, and their children, in descending age order, William, Frederik and Roland.

The initial session was with Joanna and Jonathan. By seeing the parents without their child, there is an opportunity to begin to develop the session structure with the core principles and to clarify their overall intention for themselves and for their child. I feel it is the first step in developing layers of support in their family. As all of the children came for sessions, it was possible to share and model the core principles with them, providing a framework that could be referred to by Joanna and Jonathan.

Frederik had been suffering with some physical symptoms, which required medical tests and minor operations. Joanna felt that there were also stress and anxiety issues for him and that he needed additional support. Frederik is very talented and finds it a challenge not to do anything. With this combination he tended to take on so many projects that he became compressed and overwhelmed.

Jonathan has also suffered with anxiety, which came to a head with a breakdown around the time of the birth of their third child, Roland, and the death of a close relation. This meant that Joanna found she was having to take care of the family and was not receiving support for herself. Joanna also had a background of experiencing anxiety in her life.

What became apparent in the early work was the need for support so that there was space to let down, to relax and be more in a responsive relationship for the whole family. As parents, Joanna and Jonathan hold the container for their children. So it was important to support them in their relationship.

Jonathan said that he was an 'alpha male' who survived by:

'…looking for safety and avoiding fear through control and managing every situation. Trying to avoid anything that would put me under pressure. That was a difficult environment to be in. The breakthrough was recognizing that instead of creating a hermetically sealed bubble, under which everything was tense but so far so good, getting some support allowed me to say, well, let that bubble just drop. See how I can, with some support, just try and find a way to live where I wasn't binding everybody else around me to this very compressed and stressful existence.'

He felt that this was his first experience of support, and with it he found that he could drop into the care space and come out of fight and flight. As he shared: 'This allowed me to be in a different way with Joanna and the boys.'

A second part of developing support and the family container was using brief frequent eye contact with some physical contact. This was something that Joanna and Jonathan were able to take home and continue to develop. Their intention was to check in with each other in the morning and evening. They would also find time for check-ins during the day if they felt activated. Jonathan talks about how he feels as a result of this process:

'Like a giant cloud inside me… It's just a real ache of affection really… I really, really, really love it and feel blessed.

'Sometimes it's just a settled feeling. A coming out of my head. The busyness in my brain just abating… Sometimes it's just a physical calming and settling… Sometimes I find it difficult and I can't get out of my head and I realize I haven't quite shifted into relationship.'

Joanna's experience is:

'I feel it in my pelvis, really rooted and grounded. I feel I'm not alone… Sometimes when we are checking in I can have incredible insights. It's like the space opens up for me to use my skills more… I know it's safe.'

From that place they felt they could discuss what was happening for themselves, what they needed, and importantly what was happening for each of their children. They could agree how they would respond on certain issues for their children – the boundaries that they would hold together. In this way they felt supported by each other and they were able to be the parent. The second layer of support for them was provided by me.

Joanna feels that one of the things that supported Frederik when he came for therapy was that it helped him (and her) to appreciate the intensity of the extra-curricular commitments he had at school. She described how on the one hand the extra activities had given him:

> '…something he loves but equally he's always been busy and taken on things and the music and singing have always brought joy but also compression.'

With her layers of support in place, Joanna was able to connect to her inner strength to go to the school and tell the teachers that Frederik needed to withdraw from several projects he had signed up for. Joanna believes that it was necessary to help him unload his commitments. In essence, Joanna took the responsibility as the parent to put boundaries in place that Frederik at that time was not able to do for himself. Joanna describes the outcome as:

> 'We've given him foundations through your support and he's sat in your room and he's had the opportunity to recognize where he is in his body and I know that that was incredibly challenging for him.'

Jonathan felt:

> 'I think he was given permission to pause and to feel how it felt to be compressed. To settle in that place where in that moment there is nothing else and you get a tiny taste of it…he learnt a little bit to put boundaries in place and self-regulate.'

He also made the point that he feels that their children are more willing to come for support as they know their parents are supported – that they will not just 'sponge up' issues – and that their parents are able to dissipate the issues by getting support for themselves.

For self-care, Jonathan is happy to take himself off to be on his own. Perhaps some gentle stretching exercise, meditation and quiet time. It provides a 'bit of a recharge or refresh'.

Joanna gives this example about self-care for herself and how she incorporates boundary setting to create this space:

> 'For me the self-care comes up when Jonathan wants to share something with me and I'm not able to hear it at that time. I'm able to recognize that now and

say to Jonathan that just now I need to have a cup of tea, or I was just writing a letter. It's not rude, it's just it's my boundary where I am. It's great because I think that Jonathan probably knew I wasn't ready to hear him 100 per cent anyway and it's just like that murkiness has been clarified and then I feel I can breathe. I can finish what I need to do, whether it is having a cup of tea, daydreaming, whatever. That's important to me, and then I can say I'm really ready now. What is it you wanted to say? Then we can sit and talk. It is having the courage to say this is my boundary, knowing that Jonathan is okay with that, and if he isn't and has feelings about it but this is my boundary. That's important to know that there are feelings sometimes, but then I'm in a better space to hear him when I have done what I need to do. That to me is self-care.'

Joanna has used the same process of holding the boundary with her children. If for example William is calling her she will say:

'It's not okay right now, William, but I'm free at 12. So he then knows I'll be really ready to hear him at 12. Whereas when he phones me he's probably not in the right space either, but he's pushing, pushing, pushing, because something has triggered him. If I put my boundary down, that allows him to perhaps settle, then when we do come together it's a really productive conversation.'

I suggest that her 'putting the boundary down' provides William with resistance and with that resistance he is more likely to be able to orient to where he is and slow down, settle and come into relationship. I feel it is a form of *dynamic creative opposition*.

William had been coming for sessions when it was discovered he required an urgent operation. The pace of transition was rapid, and after a sequence of tests the operation took place. The focus shifted to supporting William. The layering changed slightly. Jonathan relied on Joanna connecting with me by phone for support. As he put it to me:

'I was benefiting from Joanna linking in with you for a second layer of support and was definitely aware of it. I think over that period I probably saw you certainly less than Joanna. For my part it helped me do what I had to do, knowing that we had a resource there for sure and we were able just to concentrate on showing William that we were strong.'

Joanna stayed connected with me mostly by phone. As she explains:

'That's all I held onto were the calls. I can't remember seeing you for the two weeks that we were there. I think it was the calls that were remarkable in keeping me present.

'I didn't feel alone at any point because I knew I could call you and that if you were busy you would tell me and we would schedule a time when you

LIVERPOOL JOHN MOORES UNIVERSITY
LEARNING SERVICES

could see me. Even just making the call, it was enough to help me settle. Even though the proper call was coming perhaps half an hour later.'

As part of their support for William one of them remained with him almost all of the time. Jonathan and Joanna were able to close the boundary around the family. Jonathan recalls that they had the ability between them to be there for William in a really settled, strong and focused way. They were able to maintain their regular check-ins by taking some time together for a few minutes in the hospital corridors or possibly in a local tea room. Jonathan refers to it as 'a renewal of resource'.

Joanna points out that everything is very quick in the hospital. This created a challenge for William. As she says:

> '…working with you at that pace gave me the confidence to slow things down for William when it was getting quite tense. You could clearly see he was doing his best but he was terrified. Just by slowing someone else down in the room, giving William the opportunity to do things in his own time, gave him some courage to see it through.'

Slowing down what was happening in the room can arise out of using the pause, or also one or both parents just settling in themselves.

Joanna concludes her experience during this time with:

> 'Even with all my skills there is no way I could've done that unsupported. I could tell by my physical sensations when I was going into overwhelm: with how I was managing the situation or supporting Jonathan or William. When I would touch on a place that was too much I would then seek your support. My memory of the calls was a lot around the inner child. She was so terrified that actually all that was needed was for her to feel settled, then for me then to come back and be the wise woman, so to speak, and come into the room again.'

Indications of non-traumatized and traumatized neonates[5]

From his research work at the BEBA clinic, Castellino developed a list of characteristics, behaviours and abilities of newborns that can provide indications of whether they are traumatized or not (Castellino 1996a). I have provided a selection below from the list. The complete list is available in Appendix B.

---

5   Also known as newborns.

Characteristics, behaviours and abilities of the non-traumatized neonate

- Eyes are clear and present
- Moro and startle response is present with clear and present danger only
- Deliberate response to near or direct touch
- Crying corresponds to need
- Vibrant skin colour.

Subtle energetic, fluid tide and cranial characteristics of non-traumatized neonates are:

- Full palpable energy field with distinct clear boundaries
- Free flow of vital energy throughout the body
- Round, full cranium, absence of cranial moulding.

Shock affect characteristics in neonates

Gross observable shock in the neonate is indicated by the following:

- Glossed-over eyes
- Tactile sensitivity to near or direct touch
- Weak, hollow or empty crying sounds
- High-pitched crying sounds
- Crying inconsolably, getting lost in their emotions without ability to make visual, auditory or tactile contact
- Lack of skin colour
- Total or partial inability to orient to visual, auditory and tactile stimuli
- Generalized, or body area specific, hypotonicity.

Subtle energetic, fluid tide and cranial shock affect indicators are:

- Erratic energy field patterns

- Unresolved cranial moulding

- Weak potency within vital fluid tide

- Cranial strain patterns.

CASE STUDY: FIRST AID SKILLS[6]

Ideally as therapists it is useful to have a full case history and develop relationship as time progresses with our clients. However, there are times when that is not possible, and this case demonstrates how effective this work can be. I am grateful to the family for their permission to share their story.

I was visiting a friend who had a young family staying with them. I had been busy in another part of the house and wondered where everyone was. I could hear some cries at the top of the house. When I arrived there, there was a group of three adults including the father, Michael. They were gathered around the mother, Lisa, and her toddler daughter, Georgina, who were sitting side by side at the top of the stairs. Both were in distress and crying. Georgina's eyes had rolled back and Lisa was also in a state of serious overwhelm. Lisa was making rapid and agitated movements with her hand as she touched Georgina. Rather than connecting I sensed more of a disconnection: connection was lost between them and with the other adults around them.

My first step was to pause, take care of myself and be present: use the Mid-space exercise to ground, be aware of my body, my midline expanding to my midspace, and to settle.

I was able to gain some information as to what had happened from Lisa and the others present. In clarifying it later with Lisa she shared that:

> 'I was with Georgina in our flat. She had a high temperature which caused her to have a convulsive seizure. I was screaming in panic, could not cope and called 999.[7] This was the first time this had happened.'

I spoke first with Georgina and then to Lisa to let them know that I was here and that they were safe. Lisa had her eyes open, and after we made eye contact I asked her to look around and see where she was. Then to take a breath and notice how that felt. As she did that she began to settle a little.

6　Strategies for working with babies and parents are also discussed in Chapter 12.

7　UK Emergency Service.

I then spoke with Georgina, saying that her mum was beside her, and that it was her mum's hand touching her. I let her know where she was and that she was safe now.

Occasionally I would look around to make brief eye contact with the adults in the surround.

Each time Lisa or Georgina shifted to a more resourced place I named it to them. As they were placing their attention more with the resources they became more settled and more in relationship. As Georgina's eyes rolled back to normal, I said once more that her mum was beside her. She turned to her mum and they made eye contact. Lisa was able to hold Georgina and they continued to settle together with some support. The ambulance took them to hospital and kept them in overnight as a precaution. They were perceived to be fine so were discharged the following day.

With the development of the PPN work I would in hindsight have added some extra steps. Bringing in the two-layer support, I would have made use of the group of adults; one of them could have given some physical support to Lisa, perhaps at her back, so it would support her to relax, deepen and let down. The other adults are part of the surround of this group dynamic and I would invite them to make brief frequent eye contact and some physical contact with each other.

The cycle of pre- and perinatal therapy

To close this chapter, I would like to explore the 'cycle' of pre- and perinatal therapy work. Figure 8.1 shows the circle of life in relation to the creation of new generations. The point to consider here is that where there is healing at any stage in the cycle, it will have an effect on the other parts of the cycle.

How we grow and develop relationships during our lives can continue to be affected by the trauma imprints created in our early existence. How we are at each stage of life affects future lives. For example, the imprints held by each of the parents-to-be (which may have originated many generations earlier) are in the environment or *surround* for the foetus and infant. We have learned that where parents can develop their coherent narrative and integrate their history, their trauma imprints – adaptations – are less likely to be passed on to their child. They have the opportunity to give their child something they (the parents) did not get for themselves. The outcome is the possibility of a clearer start in life for the child and increased likelihood of developing secure attachment. Siegel (2010, p.63)[8] confirms that:

> Research reveals that the best predictor of a child's attachment is actually how a parent has made sense of his or her own early life history.

Pre- and perinatal therapy was developed to meet a need for healing early life trauma in relationship within the family system. It has also been found useful in other walks of life, such as within social and work-based relationships. Relationships work best when they come from a responsive space rather than out of survival. As we heal our trauma history, we increase our capacity to communicate from our truth; from our authentic self.

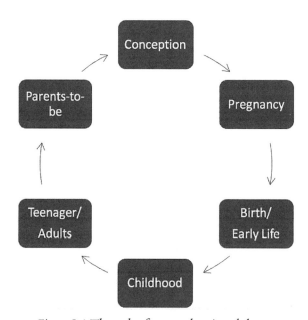

Figure 8.1 The cycle of pre- and perinatal therapy

Whilst I have primarily considered support and integration during early life, the core principles and structure can be used at any period of life. This is due to it being based on perhaps the most vulnerable period of our lives, necessitating a level of pacing and safety required to support integration and secure attachment. For this reason, although PPN therapy was developed to work in the very early stages of life and with young families, it can also be effective right through our lives.

---

8   Dozier *et al.* (2001) referred to by Siegel.

Conclusion

As we make sense of our histories and are able to differentiate our past sensations and feelings from our present-day life, our brain shifts to a more integrated, yet differentiated, social relationship with itself. The differentiation of our ancestral and current early life history from today means that we give children and ourselves the opportunity to have a clearer sense of who we truly are.

As this clarification develops within our generation, and within future generations, we get to develop a more relational society and world rather than a dysfunctional, reactive society.

I mentioned earlier about the pitfalls of too much information coming at us. Within this chapter and the previous one there is a lot of information. The essence of this form of pre- and perinatal work is about the embodiment of it. It cannot be gleaned just by reading about it. As part of honouring the work, I ask that you take the text in these two chapters as part of developing your awareness in this field. If your intention is to practise this form of therapy, I strongly recommend that you take the training in it, as well as experiencing the process workshops. In this way there is the opportunity to embody the work, to 'get it' at the somatic or felt sense level. If we attempt to work at the information level only in this field we will miss what our clients, be they adults, children, babies or even prenates, are trying to show us.

Acknowledgements for Chapters 7 and 8

Writing these two chapters has been a journey and I have been fortunate for the generous layers of support made available to me.

I want to thank Ray Castellino for creating this form of work and for his generosity in giving me permission to have carte blanche use of his material. He, together with Mary Jackson, have given their time for interviews and to answer the various questions that continued to arise.

I would also like to thank Klaus Käppeli and Regina Bücher for taking time to read the drafts and provide welcome clarifications. Also, my thanks to John Chitty for his support.

The fullness of the writing would not have been possible without the generous support of my clients. A general thank you to all my clients from whom I have learned so much. Specifically, I want to acknowledge and thank those who gave generously of their time to be interviewed and who gave permission to include their stories. For the reason of confidentiality, I am not saying who, but you each know who you are and I thank you.

References for Chapters 7 and 8

BEBA (2016) *About Early Trauma.* Santa Barbara, CA: BEBA. Available at http://beba.org/early-traum, accessed on 7 October 2016.

Buss, C., Davis, E.P., Shahbaba, B., Pruessner, J.C., Head, K., and Sandman, C.A. (2012) 'Maternal cortisol over the course of pregnancy and subsequent child amygdala and hippocampus volumes and affective problems.' *Proceedings of the National Academy of Sciences 109*, 20, E1312–E1319.

Caldji, C., Diorio, J., and Meaney, M.J. (2000) 'Variations in maternal care in infancy regulate the development of stress reactivity.' *Biological Psychiatry 48*, 12, 1164–1174.

Castellino, R. (1996a) *Being with Newborns: An Introduction to Somatotropic Therapy; Attention to the Newborn; Healing Betrayal, New Hope for the Prevention of Violence.* Santa Barbara, CA: Castellino Training.

Castellino, R. (1996b) *The Polarity Therapy Paradigm Regarding Pre-Conception, Prenatal and Birth Imprinting.* Santa Barbara, CA: Castellino Training.

Castellino, R. (2014) *Two Layers of Support – Creating the Conditions for Healing.* DVD. London: Whole Being Films.

Castellino, R. (2015a) *Module 3 Foundation Training. Vaginal Birth: Birth Stages, Pelvic Types and Cranial Molding Course Notes.* Santa Barbara, CA: Castellino Training.

Castellino, R. (2015b) *The Relational Rhythm and Blueprint.* Private interview with Ray Castellino DC (retired). RPP, RCST.

Castellino, R. (2015c) *Womb Surround Process Workshop Manual.* Santa Barbara, CA: Castellino Training.

Castellino, R., Jackson, M., and Blasco, T.M. (2013–2017) *Castellino Foundation Training in Pre- and Perinatal Therapy.* Santa Barbara, CA: Castellino Training.

Chamberlain, D.B. (2006) 'About real babies.' *Journal of Prenatal & Perinatal Psychology & Health 21*, 2, 111–115.

Colman, A.M. (2015) *Oxford Dictionary of Psychology.* Oxford, UK: Oxford University Press. (Updated 2016.)

DiPietro, J.A., Novak, M.F.S.X., Costigan, K.A., Atella, L.D., and Reusing, S.P. (2006) 'Maternal psychological distress during pregnancy in relation to child development at age two.' *Child Development 77*, 3, 573–587.

Dodd, V.L. (2005) 'Implications of kangaroo care for growth and development in preterm infants.' *Journal of Obstetric, Gynecologic, & Neonatal Nursing 34*, 2, 218–232.

Dozier, M.K., Stovall, C., Albus, K.E., and Bates, B. (2001) 'Attachment for infants in foster care: The role of caregiver state of mind.' *Child Development 72*, 5, 1467–1477.

Emerson, W.R. (1996) 'The vulnerable prenate.' *Pre- and Perinatal Psychology 10*, 3, 18.

Field, T. (1985) *Attachment as a Psychobiological Attunement: Being on the Same Wavelength in the Psychobiology of Attachment and Separation.* Orlando, FL: Academic Press.

Gabriel, M. (1992) *Voices from the Womb: Adults Re-live Their Pre-birth Experiences.* Lower Lake, CA: Aslan.

Gerhardt, S. (2015) *Why Love Matters: How Affection Shapes a Baby's Brain.* Hove, UK: Routledge.

Grof, S. (2007) *Psychology of the Future: Lessons from Modern Consciousness Research.* Available at www.stanislavgrof.com/wp-content/uploads/pdf/Psychology_of_the_Future.pdf, accessed on 19 July 2016.

Gunnar, M., Malone, S., and Fisch, R. (1985a) 'The psychobiology of stress and coping in the human neonate: Studies of adrenocortical responses to stress in the first week of life.' *Stress and Coping 1*, 179–196.

Gunnar, M., Malone, S., Vance, G., and Fisch, R. (1985b) 'Coping with aversive stimulation in the neonatal period: Quiet sleep and plasma cortisol levels during recovery from circumcision.' *Child Development 56*, 4, 824–834.

Hanson, J.L., Chung, M.K., Avants, B.B., Shirtcliff, E.A., *et al.* (2010) 'Early stress is associated with alterations in the orbitofrontal cortex: A tensor-based morphometry investigation of brain structure and behavioral risk.' *The Journal of Neuroscience: The Official Journal of the Society for Neuroscience 30*, 22, 7466–7472.

Jackson, M. (2015) *Aspects of Birth and Pre and Perinatal Therapy.* Private interview with Mary Jackson RN, CPM, LM, RCST.

Johnson, A.N. (2005) 'Kangaroo holding beyond the NICU.' *Journal of Pediatric Nursing 31*, 1, 53–56.

Kern, M. (2001) *Wisdom in the Body.* London: Thorsons.

LeDoux, J.E. (2015) 'The amygdala is NOT the brain's fear center: Separating findings from conclusions.' *Psychology Today.* Available at https://www.psychologytoday.com/blog/i-got-mind-tell-you/201508/the-amygdala-is-not-the-brains-fear-center, accessed on 1 November 2016.

Levine, P.A. and Frederick, A. (1997) *Waking the Tiger: Healing Trauma.* Berkeley, CA: North Atlantic Books.

Levine, P.A. and Kline, M. (2007) *Trauma Through a Child's Eyes.* Berkeley, CA: North Atlantic Books.

Ludington-Hoe, S.M., and Swinth, J.Y. (1996) 'Developmental aspects of kangaroo care.' *Journal of Obstetric, Gynecologic, & Neonatal Nursing 25*, 8, 691–703.

Maslow, A. (1954) *Maslow's Hierarchy of Needs.* Available at www.businessballs.com/maslow.htm, accessed on 10 October 2016.

McEwen, B.S., Eiland, L., Hunter, R.G., and Miller, M.M. (2012) 'Stress and anxiety: Structural plasticity and epigenetic regulation as a consequence of stress.' *Neuropharmacology 62*, 1, 3–12.

McGregor, J. and Casey, J. (2012) *Enhancing Parent–Infant Bonding Using Kangaroo Care: A Structured Review.* The Royal College of Midwives: Evidence Based Midwifery, June. Available at www.rcm.org.uk/learning-and-career/learning-and-research/ebm-articles/enhancing-parent-infant-bonding-using, accessed on 10 October 2016.

Moberg, K.U. (2011) *The Oxytocin Factor: Tapping the Hormone of Calm, Love, and Healing.* London: Pinter & Martin.

Neufeld, G. and Maté, G. (2006) *Hold Onto Your Kids.* New York: Ballantine.

Ogden, P., Minton, K., and Pain, C. (2006) *Trauma and the Body: A Sensorimotor Approach to Psychotherapy.* New York: Norton.

Panksepp, J. (1998) *Affective Neuroscience: The Foundations of Human and Animal Emotions.* New York: Oxford University Press.

Panksepp, J. (2009) 'Brain Emotional Systems and Qualities of Mental Life: From Animal Models of Affect to Implications for Psychotherapeutics.' In D. Fosha, D.J. Siegel and M.F. Solomon (eds) *The Healing Power of Emotion: Affective Neuroscience, Development & Clinical Practice.* New York: Norton.

Panksepp, J. (2010) 'The Basic Affective Circuits of Mammalian Brains: Implications for Healthy Human Development and the Cultural Landscapes of ADHD.' In C.M. Worthman, P.M. Plotsky, D.S. Schechter and C.A. Cummings (eds) *Formative Experiences: The Interaction of Care-Giving, Culture, and Developmental Psychobiology.* New York: Cambridge University Press.

Panksepp, J. and Biven, L. (2012) *The Archaeology of Mind: Neuroevolutionary Origins of Human Emotions.* Norton Series on Interpersonal Neurobiology. New York: Norton.

Porges, S.W. (2011) *The Polyvagal Theory: Neurophysiological Foundations of Emotions, Attachment, Communication, and Self-Regulation.* New York: Norton.

Porges, S.W. (2013) *The Polyvagal Theory for Treating Trauma.* Transcript of interview with Ruth Buczynski. The National Institute for the Clinical Application of Behavioral Medicine.

Radley, J.J. and Morrison, J.H. (2005) 'Repeated stress and structural plasticity in the brain.' *Ageing Research Reviews 4*, 2, 271–287.

Schore, A.N. (1994) *Affect Regulation and the Origin of the Self.* Hillsdale, NJ, and Hove, UK: Lawrence Erlbaum.

Schore, A.N. (2003) *Affect Dysregulation and Disorders of the Self.* London and New York: Norton.

Siegel, D.J. (2010) *The Mindful Therapist: A Clinician's Guide to Mindsight and Neural Integration.* New York: Norton.

Siegel, D.J. (2012) *The Developing Mind: How Relationships and the Brain Interact to Shape Who We Are.* New York: Guilford.

Siegel, D.J. and Hartzell, M. (2003) *Parenting From the Inside Out.* New York: Tarcher/Putnam.

Stone, R. (1985) *Health Building: The Conscious Art of Living Well.* Sebastopol, CA: CRCS Publications.

Tronick, E. (2009) *Still Face Experiment.* University of Boston: Zero To Three. Available at www.zerotothree.org. Available at www.youtube.com/watch?v=apzXGEbZht0, accessed on 2 November 2016.

Tudor, K., Merry, T., and Dryden, W. (2002) *Dictionary of Person-centred Psychology.* London: Wiley.

Van der Kolk, B. (2014) *The Body Keeps the Score: Mind. Brain and Body in the Transformation of Trauma.* London: Penguin.

Wilbarger, P. and Wilbarger, J. (1997) *Sensory Defensiveness and Related Social/Emotional and Neurological Problems.* Van Nuys, CA: Wilbarger.

Wilks, J. (2015) *Choices in Pregnancy and Childbirth: A Guide to Options for Health Professionals, Midwives, Holistic Practitioners, and Parents.* London and Philadelphia: Singing Dragon.

Yehuda, R. (2015) *How Trauma and Resilience Cross Generations.* Radio interview, NPR One.

Yehuda, R., Daskalakis, N.P., Bierer, L.M., Bader, H.N., *et al.* (2015) 'Holocaust exposure induced intergenerational effects on FKBP5 methylation.' *Biological Psychiatry 2015.* Available at www.biologicalpsychiatryjournal.com/article/S0006-3223(15)00652-6/pdf, accessed on 10 October 2016.

CHAPTER 9

ALLERGIES, GUT HEALTH, AUTOIMMUNITY AND THE MICROBIOME

Dr Carolyn Goh

CASE STUDY

Sara, aged one year, was born at 41 weeks by Caesarean section. The surgery was straightforward and both mum and baby recovered well. Sara was breastfed. At the age of three weeks Sara started displaying the typical signs of colic. She would cry endlessly in the evenings and find it very difficult to settle. Her discomfort would ease if she managed to burp or pass wind. She also developed reflux. She was put on medication to manage her reflux and colic. Her symptoms subsided at about four months. At six months of age, Sara was introduced to solids. A couple of weeks later she suffered from a severe allergic reaction to eggs. She has eczema and is also allergic to peanuts. Mum suffers from irritable bowel syndrome (IBS) and Dad has eczema and a history of asthma as a child.

This is a typical medical history of a baby that I often come across in my clinic.

Atopic diseases such as atopic dermatitis, asthma and food allergies have reached epidemic proportions during the past decades in industrialized countries and, more recently, in developing countries. What is responsible for the increasing rate of atopic conditions seen in children?

Genetic predisposition, in the form of filaggrin[1] gene mutations (Palmer *et al.* 2006), was thought to be the fundamental factor governing

---

1   Filaggrin plays an important role in the skin's barrier function.

susceptibility to atopic disease and allergy. However, the rise in atopy has occurred within too short a time frame to be explained by a genetic shift in the population, thus pointing to environmental or lifestyle changes. Although some increase in exposure to allergens to sensitize and then trigger attacks has been observed (such as increased exposure to house dust mites in modern, centrally heated houses), these changes do not seem to adequately explain this exponential rise (Bloomfield *et al.* 2006). This has led to the search for other factors to explain this phenomenon.

One theory is the hygiene hypothesis, formulated in 1989 by an epidemiologist, David Strachan (Strachan 1989), who reported an inverse relationship between family size and development of atopic disorders, and proposed that a lower incidence of infection in early childhood (e.g. due to a lack of unhygienic contact with older siblings or acquired prenatally) could be a cause of the rise in allergic diseases. Subsequently, as the concept was further explored by specialists in allergy and immunology, it evolved into the broader notion that declining microbial exposure is a major causative factor in the increasing incidence of atopy in recent years. A wide range of factors which might have resulted in altered microbial exposure have been examined, such as clean water and food, sanitation, antibiotics and vaccines, and birth practices, as well as incidental factors such as the move from countryside to urban living (Bloomfield *et al.* 2006).

Research carried out by the Human Microbiome Project (n.d.) is showing us that microbial exposure is the key to developing a healthy microbiome population which in turn determines our susceptibility to disease as well as health in general. Ninety per cent of the cells in our body are microbacteria and 99 per cent of our genome is made up of the microbiome (Human Microbiome Project n.d.). So, we really are ruled by our microbes. These microbes play a huge role in helping us develop from birth and determine our health as adults. It is therefore essential that the microbes that inhabit our bodies are the right ones!

The population of microbes that we play host to is dependent on our exposure to these microbes throughout life. Term and preterm infants were thought to be born essentially sterile, but new evidence of bacterial translocation in utero (Jiménez *et al.* 2005) and the presence of microbial life in preterm infants' meconium (Ardissone *et al.* 2014) refute this. Observed lipopolysaccharide (LPS), an endotoxin of Gram-negative bacteria in the cord blood of preterm infants, provides evidence of the translocation process in utero (Martinez-Lopez *et al.* 2014). The health of our early microbial population pre-birth is therefore largely determined by the health of the maternal microbial population during pregnancy.

The role of microbes

Research (Jašarević *et al.* 2015) shows that stress plays a huge role in the health and population of microbes that live in us. Maternal stress levels can cause a shift in microbial population which are then passed on to the baby. Researchers utilized an established mouse model of early maternal stress, which included intervals of exposure to a predator odour, restraint and novel noise as stressors. Two days after birth, tissue was collected from the mothers using vaginal lavages and maternal faecal pellets and offspring distal gut were analysed. Offspring brains were examined to measure transport of amino acids. Researchers found that stress during pregnancy was associated with disruption of maternal vaginal and offspring gut microbiota composition (Jašarević *et al.* 2015).

Babies also acquire microbes from the birth canal of the mother during birth. Healthy microbes found in the mother's birth canal are passed on to populate the gut of the baby. These microbes influence multiple processes including the differentiation of epithelium, cross-talk within the gut-associated lymphoid tissue (GALT), gastrointestinal tract morphology, nutrition and metabolism (Cebra 1999; Cho and Blaser 2012; Guaraldi and Salvatori 2012; Hooper, Littman and Macpherson 2012; Putignani *et al.* 2014). A normal, healthy vaginal delivery introduces vaginal microbes, which helps set the bar for immune reactions and is responsible for maturation of the GALT (Weng and Walker 2013). The development of a normal infant gut and the immune system requires interaction between intestinal epithelial cells, lymphoid tissue and microbiomes. These microbiomes are believed to maintain a state of regulated inflammation that is important in providing cross-talk between microbes of the intestinal epithelium (Neu 2007) and the GALT (Weng and Walker 2013). Apoptotic stimuli, reactive oxygen synthesis and Toll-like receptor (TLR) signalling are induced by the microbes to produce a state of controlled inflammation that helps develop the innate immune defences and promotes pathogen recognition (Jakaitis and Denning 2014; Kaplan, Shi and Walker 2011). The developing commensal microbiota alters gut microanatomy and function by promoting epithelial turnover and synthesis of mucus, increasing peristalsis, which decreases small intestinal colonization, and secreting various antimicrobial compounds in the mucus (Adlerberth and Wold 2009; Johansson, Sjovall and Hansson 2013). These interactions enable the infant gut to quickly develop tolerance to food antigens and the commensal microbiota, and provides a barrier against penetration of pathogenic microbes into the mucosa and submucosa (Groer *et al.* 2014).

If, however, the maternal microbiome is unhealthy, this will pass on to the baby, which in turn will develop a population of unhealthy microbes. These microbes are not primed to carry out the functions such as digestive development and immune system maturity. The baby is then predisposed to digestive problems such as colic and atopic conditions.

The gut–brain connection

Gut microbes have also been associated with the early development of the nervous system. Microbes can communicate with the brain via the vagus nerve (Field and Diego 2008). The brain and the gut bacteria have constant cross-talk through what is known as the microbiome–gut–brain axis via the vagus nerve as well as through the release of neurochemicals (Dockray 2014). This extension of the gut–brain axis to include the microbiome results in the microbiota–gut–brain axis. This axis represents a complex network of communication between the gut, intestinal microbiota and the brain, modulating immune, GI and CNS functions, and encompasses the CNS, SNS and PSNS branches of the ANS as well as the enteric nervous system (Borre *et al.* 2014; Grenham *et al.* 2011).

The microbiota–gut–brain axis plays a huge role in the neurodevelopmental phases. Studies on germ-free mice have shown that bacterial colonization of the gut is central to the development and maturation of both the ENS and CNS (Barbara *et al.* 2005; Stiling, Dinan and Cryan 2014). In childhood and adolescence early colonization and microbiome development can determine general as well as mental health in later life (Diaz Heijtz *et al.* 2011; Theije, Worperisis and Ramadan 2014).

The vagus and the microbiome

The vagus nerve is the parasympathetic output of the brain and serves to provide motor function to the digestive tract. Reduction of output of the vagus nerve results in sluggish intestinal activity. In the newborn, this sluggishness can result in constipation and colic as well as inflammation.

Vagal tone, a marker of active functioning of the vagus nerve, is necessary for the development of the nervous system and brain (Field and Diego 2008). Reduced vagal tone is one of the best indicators of neurologic health of a newborn, and poor vagal tone is associated with social, behavioural, emotional and communication problems later in life and failure to grow and gain weight (Porges 2011). Microbes also produce the neurochemicals dopamine and serotonin that affect behaviour, and studies (Neufeld *et al.* 2011; Sudo *et al.* 2004) have shown that specific microbes can reduce anxiety in normal, healthy rodents.

Stephen Porges[2] talks about the hierarchy and development of our nervous system (see Chapter 3). At birth, babies do not have a fully developed nervous system. They exhibit a lower vagal tone which increases as they develop. Studies by Porges (e.g. Doussard-Roosevelt *et al.* 1997) have shown that vagal tone in babies is reduced below three months of age, and in some babies right up until six months of age. This has a profound effect on how the nervous system responds to situations and stimuli. When vagal tone is low, this means that the ability of the nervous system to 'correct' itself when it goes out of balance is hampered. Perhaps the communication of microbes with the brain via the vagus nerve stimulates vagus activity and aids in the development of vagal tone. It is known, for example, that probiotic bacteria such as *Lactobacillus rhamnosus* stimulate vagal function, resulting in improved weight gain and brain function (Perez-Birgos *et al.* 2013).

The vagus nerve is an important, though apparently not the only, mediator of microbiota–gut–brain interaction and may depend on the bacterial strain used. Altered gut motility or neuroactive signals secreted by bacteria could result in an increased or decreased activation of the vagal pathway (Barbara *et al.* 2005). The exact modalities of how the vagus interacts with the microbiota to induce such effects remain unclear. More research in the development of the nervous system and the microbiome

---

2   Emeritus Professor of Psychiatry at the University of Illinois at Chicago and developer of the Polyvagal Theory.

needs to be carried out to determine how altered vagal activation leads to sustainable epigenetic modifications in the dorsal nucleus of the vagus nerve.

How birth affects the microbiome

A baby born by Caesarean section receives microbes such as *Staphylococcus*, *Corynebacterium* and *Propionibacterium spp* from skin contact and touch (Dominguez-Bello *et al.* 2010). However, these microbes may not be primed to help in the development of the baby's immune system, nervous system or maturity of the digestive process. The immune system may not be configured correctly, causing inappropriate immune reactions associated with an increased risk of atopic diseases such as asthma, eczema, allergic rhinitis and allergies to food. Research by Biasucci *et al.* (2008) showed that the gut microbiota after Caesarean delivery was characterized by an absence of *Bifidobacteria* species, which are thought to be important to the postnatal development of the immune system, whereas vaginally delivered neonates showed a predominance of these species. In addition, Caesarean-born children also tend to have delayed access to breast milk, which has a potent influence on gut microbiota (Mead 2008). Caesarean-section babies also tend to be more susceptible to infections and illnesses which often result in the consumption of broad-spectrum antibiotics, which effectively wipes out whatever population of bacteria they did acquire.

Dr Maria Gloria Dominguez-Bello, associate professor in the Human Microbiome Program at the NYU School of Medicine, runs a programme to use vaginal swabs to populate the microbes in babies born by Caesarean section (Human Microbiome Program n.d.). The mothers are screened ensuring they are HIV-negative and strep-B negative, and have an acid, lactobacillus-dominated vagina. In an interview in 2014 Dr Dominguez-Bello says the initial findings so far suggest that using gauze to gather a mother's birth-canal bacteria and then impart them to babies born by C-section does make those babies' bacterial populations more closely resemble vaginally born babies, though only partially (Dominguez-Bello 2014).

She explains that, during labour, the baby is rubbing against the mucosa of the birth canal for a long time and bacteria start growing and colonizing the baby during birth exponentially. Labour is an important part of the colonization process. Antibiotics are routinely prescribed during Caesarean sections and this could be another reason for partial repopulation.

Breastfeeding vs bottle-feeding

Other factors that determine the population of microbes colonizing babies are breast or bottle feeding, Mum's diet, microbes from Dad, and early and extensive bathing. Breastfeeding plays a huge part in determining the population of microbes in the baby's gut. In full-term infants, the species of microbes that colonize the early gut differ between those who are breast-fed compared with formula-fed infants (Bezirtzoglou, Tsiotsias and Welling 2011). There are more than 200 HMOs (Human Milk Oligosaccharides) found in breast milk, the third largest component behind lactose and fat (Newburg 2013). HMOs are indigestible by the infant, and remain largely intact during passage to the colon, where they are then broken down into short-chain fatty acids by intestinal microbiota that promote the growth of *Bifidobacteria* and *Lactobacillus* (De Leoz *et al.* 2015; Martin and Sela 2013). The *Bifidobacterium longum infantis* strain can digest HMOs with incredible efficiency, eating all the available food and increasing its population. This makes it harder for pathogens to establish themselves (Underwood *et al.* 2015). The HMOs also deter these invaders more directly. Many pathogens launch their invasions by first recognizing sugar molecules on the surface of intestinal cells. HMOs resemble those sugars, and so act like floating decoys that draw pathogens away from the gut itself. So, breast milk selects for beneficial microbes while also warding off harmful ones (Turroni *et al.* 2014). It sets babies up with the right pioneers.

Formula-fed infant faeces contain higher numbers of *Atopobium*, lower numbers of *Bifidobacterium*, and an increased relative abundance of *Bacteroides* (Bezirtzoglou *et al.* 2011). Interestingly, when breast-fed babies receive mixed feeding of both human milk and formula, the microbiota shifts to a community structure that more closely resembles that found in formula-fed infants, which is similar to when the infants begin solid food (Guaraldi and Salvatori 2012). This 'formula/solid food' microbiome is dominated by *Enterococci* and *Enterobacteria, Bacteroides, Clostridia* and other anaerobic *Streptococci* (Guaraldi and Salvatori 2012). Interestingly, milk from preterm mothers is different in many ways from that produced by term mothers. For example, preterm milk appears to have a different mix of HMOs that could influence microbial growth (De Leoz *et al.* 2012). Perhaps they serve a different function and are needed for development at this early stage.

Breastfeeding can also help control the population of unhealthy maternal microbes that have been passed down. If a mother is breastfeeding, antibodies against the unhealthy antigens in the body will be passed to the baby through breast milk. These will help to control the baby's unhealthy population of gut flora. Once breastfeeding stops, the protection is removed and the unhealthy gut flora repopulate. This could be one of the reasons why mothers notice a rise in ear infections and general ill health once breastfeeding stops (Campbell-McBride 2010).

The development of the microbiome

How does the early gut microbiome develop into the adult gut microbiome and what factors could influence the process? The Human Microbiome Project carried out a study (Lozupone *et al.* 2013) using samples of microbes that were taken from different body sites of different adults. The developmental trajectory of one infant's gut from birth (where it resembles the mother's vaginal community) over the first two and a half years of life was mapped onto these samples (Koenig *et al.* 2011). By two and a half years it resembled the adult gut. An interesting observation was that when the baby was given antibiotics, the trajectory regressed (Koenig *et al.* 2011). The microbiome did recover, but the effect this could have on the developing microbiome and impact on health in later life is yet to be discovered. Recent statistics from the CDC report that, in one year, 262.5 million courses of antibiotics are written in the outpatient setting, equating to more than five prescriptions written each year for every six people in the United States (Hicks *et al.* 2015).

The early microbiome is likely to determine the signature of the adult microbiome, based on the founder effect, whereby the original colonizing microbiota are instrumental in the direction of the assemblage. As a result, the initial colonizing of microbiota is likely to be a critical determinant in the development of certain paediatric diseases (Nieuwdorp *et al.* 2014). The early microbiota produces active metabolites such as folate, butyrate and acetate, which could epigenetically alter gut epithelium and hepatic and immune cells, a type of developmental programming which might later translate into risks for a variety of human diseases, including obesity (Mischke and Plosch 2013).

It is important to get these first communities right. They steer the development of the immune system, creating a balanced set of sentries that can detect and respond to pathogens, without also going berserk at innocuous triggers such as pollen or dust. However, it is never too late to start creating a diverse and healthy population of microbes. Nutrition is a major factor in helping to maintain and develop a healthy, prosperous garden of good microbes.

The GAPS approach

In the Gut and Psychology Syndrome (GAPS), Dr Natasha Campbell-McBride (2010) observed the connection between the health of the gut and mental as well as physiological diseases in her work as a neurologist. She recommends a nutritional protocol to help heal the gut and create a healthy microbial population. Some of her recommendations for babies and children are described here.

Bottle-fed and breast-fed babies should be introduced to solids from the age of four months and six months respectively. Solids should be introduced gradually, starting from just one very small meal a day with the rest of the meals being breast milk or formula with some probiotic added. A note of caution when using probiotics for infants is that it can cause diarrhoea and/or constipation. Be sure to use an infant probiotic.

The first week of introduction of solids should consist of meat stock. Chicken stock is particularly gentle on the stomach. Freshly pressed vegetable or fruit juice mixed with some warm water between meals can be introduced. Refrain from giving any commercially available vegetable or fruit juices. Vegetable soup or puree from peeled, de-seeded and well-cooked vegetables (non-starch vegetables, so no potato, sweet potato, yams or parsnips) can be introduced in the second week. This can be followed by boiled meats (cooked for a long time in water and then pureed) added into the baby's vegetable soups and puree in the third week. Carry on topping up the baby's meals with breast milk if breastfeeding. On week four you can start introducing egg by adding raw organic egg yolk (a quarter teaspoon) into his or her vegetable puree. Watch for any reaction. If there is none, gradually increase the amount of raw egg yolk and start adding it to every bowl of soup or vegetable puree.

For more information on the types of vegetables, meats and fruit, how they should be prepared and the nutritional protocol for weeks 1–10, refer to GAPS (n.d.).

A good indication of a baby's sensitivity to a particular food is the consistency of his or her stool. Loose stool, diarrhoea or constipation are an indication of a sensitivity to a new food being introduced. Remove it from the diet, wait for a few weeks, then try to introduce it again. Another common reaction is a new skin rash or an eczema flare-up.

It is also advised that babies should not be exposed to harsh chemicals. Try using natural products to clean the home, natural detergents for laundry and avoid taking a baby to chlorinated swimming pools, hospitals and newly redecorated places. Babies do not need to be cleaned or washed with any soap or shampoo. Use clean, warm water. Soaps wash off protective oils from the baby's skin and expose it to drying out and invasion by pathogens. Breast milk works very well for any skin condition such as acne, rash and nappy rash and even ear infections. Coconut and olive oil are also very good skin moisturizers.

Children are advised to consume meat broths, fresh vegetable and fruit juices as well as fermented foods. Processed foods, sugar and additives should not be consumed. Children experiencing digestive issues such as diarrhoea and abdominal pain should go on the more restrictive GAPS Introduction Diet (GAPS n.d.) in order to heal the gut and encourage growth of healthy microbes.

Supplements such as fermented cod liver oil, essential fatty acids and a therapeutic grade probiotic are also recommended. However, the main treatment protocol is based on nutrition and, as such, supplements are not essential. Proper nutrition is the stepping stone to a healthy garden of microbes and is essential to ensure a healthy immune and nervous system. Research on the microbiome and its importance has led to numerous brands of probiotic products, each with their own individual composition of microbes, being made available to the consumer. In my opinion, care should be taken when choosing a probiotic and it should be taken with the advice of a nutritionist or qualified therapist. We are still unsure of the exact composition of microbes in the healthy gut and this varies from person to person. It may be a little presumptuous to assume that consuming a microbe that is not meant to live in us can do no harm. Consumption of microbes via fermented foods is a much safer way of introducing microbes into our body as they pass through every stage of our digestive system. The natural selection process of the body using enzymes and acidity levels ensures that the right microbes are housed in the right areas.

The mounting knowledge on the microbiome and its role in the development of our immune and nervous systems is changing the way we see and treat medical conditions from schizophrenia to obesity. This will play a big role in propelling necessary changes to our dietary habits, birthing and after-care of babies and children as well as the use of antibiotics. Nutrition, especially in mums-to-be, babies and children, is extremely important in ensuring a good, healthy start to life, and therapists of all kinds have an important role in pointing parents in the right direction to good quality advice.

The GAPS protocol has been used very successfully with autistic children who almost always have gut issues. The jury is still out on a definite cause for autism and although vaccination is sometimes singled out as one of the contributing factors, studies done by Shultz et al. (2008) and Shaw (2013) raised the question whether regression into autism is triggered, not by the measles-mumps-rubella (MMR) vaccine, but by acetaminophen (paracetamol) found in Calpol and Tylenol given routinely for fever and pain. In his latest paper, Schultz (2016) recommends that acetaminophen use be reviewed for safety in children due to dysfunction of the endocannabinoid system which leads to ASD (see Appendix C).

References

Adlerberth, I. and Wold, A.E. (2009) 'Establishment of the gut microbiota in Western infants.' *Acta Paediatr. 98*, 229–238.

Ardissone, A.N., De la Cruz, D.M., Davis-Richardson, A.G., Rechcigl, K.T., *et al.* (2014) 'Meconium microbiome analysis identifies bacteria correlated with premature birth.' *PLoS One 9*, e90784.

Barbara, G., Stanghellini, V., Brandi, G., Cremon, C., *et al.* (2005) 'Interactions between commensal bacteria and gut sensorimotor function in health and disease.' *Am. J. Gastroenterol. 100*, 11, 2560–2568.

Bezirtzoglou, E., Tsiotsias, A., and Welling, G.W. (2011) 'Microbiota profile in feces of breast- and formula-fed newborns by using fluorescence in situ hybridization (FISH). *Anaerobe 17*, 478–482.

Biasucci, G., Benenati, B., Morelli, L., Bessi, E., and Boehm, G. (2008) 'Cesarean delivery may affect the early biodiversity of intestinal bacteria.' *J. Nutr. 138*, 9, 1796S–1800S.

Bloomfield, S.F., Stanwell-Smith, R., Crevel, R.W.R., and Pickup, J. (2006) 'Too clean, or not too clean: The Hygiene Hypothesis and home hygiene.' *Clin. Exp. Allergy 36*, 4, 402–425.

Borre, Y.E., O'Keeffe, G.W., Clarke, G., Stanton, C., Dinan, T.G., and Cryan, J.F. (2014) 'Microbiota and neurodevelopmental windows: Implications for brain disorders.' *Trends Mol. Med. 20*, 9, 509–518.

Campbell-McBride, N. (2010) *Gut and Psychology Syndrome: Natural Treatment for Autism, Dyspraxia, ADD, Dyslexia, ADHD, Depression, Schizophrenia*. Wymondham, Norfolk: Medinform Publishing.

Cebra, J.J. (1999) 'Influences of microbiota on intestinal immune system development.' *Am. J. Clin. Nutr. 69*, 1046S–1051S.

Cho, I. and Blaser, M.J. (2012) 'The human microbiome: At the interface of health and disease.' *Nat. Rev. Genet. 13*, 260–270.

De Leoz, M.L., Gaerlan, S.C., Strum, J.S., Dimapasoc, L.M., *et al.* (2012) 'Lacto-N-tetraose, fucosylation, and secretor status are highly variable in human milk oligosaccharides from women delivering preterm.' *J. Proteome Res. 11*, 4662–4672.

De Leoz, M.L., Kalanetra, K.M., Bokulich, N.A., Strum, J.S. *et al.* (2015) 'Human milk glycomics and gut microbial genomics in infant feces shows correlation between human milk oligosaccharides and gut microbiota: A proof of concept study.' *J. Proteome Res. 14*, 491–502.

Diaz Heijtz, R., Wang, S., Anuar, F., Qian, Y., *et al.* (2011) 'Normal gut microbiota modulates brain development and behavior.' *Proc. Natl. Acad. Sci. USA 108*, 7, 3047–3052.

Dockray, G.J. (2014) 'Gastrointestinal hormones and the dialogue between gut and brain.' *J. Physiol. 592 (Pt 14)*, 2927–2941.

Dominguez-Bello, M.G. (2014) *Could Birth-Canal Bacteria Help C-Section Babies?* Common Health. Available at www.wbur.org/commonhealth/2014/06/25/birth-canal-bacteria-c-section, accessed on 10 October 2016.

Dominguez-Bello, M.G., Costello, E.K., Contreras, M., Magris, M., *et al.* (2010) 'Delivery mode shapes the acquisition and structure of the initial microbiota across multiple body habitats in newborns.' *Proc. Natl. Acad. Sci. USA 107*, 26, 11971–11975.

Doussard-Roosevelt, J., Porges, S., Scanlon, J., Alemi, B., and Scanlon, K. (1997) 'Vagal regulation of heart rate in the prediction of developmental outcome for very low birth weight preterm infants.' *Child Development 68*, 173–186.

Field, T. and Diego, M. (2008) 'Vagal activity, early growth and emotional development.' *Infant Behav. Dev. 31*, 3, 361–373.

GAPS (n.d.) *Gut and Psychology Syndrome.* Available at www.gaps.me, accessed on 10 October 2016.

Grenham, S., Clarke, G., Cryan, J.F., and Dinan, T.G. (2011) 'Brain–gut–microbe communication in health and disease.' *Front. Physio. 2*, 94.

Groer, M.W., Luciano, A.A., Dishaw, L.J., Ashmeade, T.L., Miller, E., and Gilbert, J.A. (2014) 'Development of the preterm infant gut microbiome: A research priority.' *Microbiome 2*, 38.

Guaraldi, F. and Salvatori, G. (2012) 'Effect of breast and formula feeding on gut microbiota shaping in newborns.' *Front. Cell Infect. Microbiol. 2*, 94.

Hicks, L.A., Bartoces, M.G., Roberts, R.M., Suda, K.J., *et al.* (2015) 'U.S. outpatient antibiotic prescribing variation according to geography, patient population, and provider specialty in 2011.' *Clin. Infect. Dis. 60*, 9, 1308–1316.

Hooper, L.V., Littman, D.R., and Macpherson, A.J. (2012) 'Interactions between the microbiota and the immune system.' *Science 336*, 1268–1273.

Human Microbiome Project (n.d.). Available at http://hmpdacc.org, accessed on 10 October 2016.

Jakaitis, B.M. and Denning, P.W. (2014) 'Commensal and probiotic bacteria may prevent NEC by maturing intestinal host defenses.' *Pathophysiology 21*, 47–54.

Jašarević, E., Howerton, C.L., Howard, C.D., and Bale, T.L. (2015) 'Alterations in the vaginal microbiome by maternal stress are associated with metabolic reprogramming of the offspring gut and brain.' *Endocrinology 56*, 9, 3265–3276.

Jiménez, E., Fernández, L., Marín, M.L., Martín, R., *et al.* (2005) 'Isolation of commensal bacteria from umbilical cord blood of healthy neonates born by cesarean section.' *Curr. Microbiol. 51*, 4, 270–274.

Johansson, M.E., Sjovall, H., and Hansson, G.C. (2013) 'The gastrointestinal mucus system in health and disease.' *Nat. Rev. Gastroenterol. Hepatol. 10*, 352–361.

Kaplan, J.L., Shi, H.N., and Walker, W.A. (2011) 'The role of microbes in developmental immunologic programming.' *Pediatr. Res. 69*, 465–472.

Koenig, J.E., Spor, A., Scalfone, N., Fricker, A.D., *et al.* (2011) 'Succession of microbial consortia in the developing infant gut microbiome.' *Proc. Natl. Acad. Sci. USA 108*, Suppl. 1, 4578–4585.

Lozupone, C.A., Stombaugh, J., Gonzalez, A., Ackermann, G., *et al.* (2013) 'Meta-analyses of studies of the human microbiota.' *Genome Res. 23*, 10, 1704–1714.

Martin, M. and Sela, D.S. (2013) 'Infant Gut Microbiota: Developmental Influences and Health Outcomes.' In K. Clancy, K. Hinde and J. Rutherford (eds) *Building Babies: Primate Development in Proximate and Ultimate Perspective.* New York: Springer.

Martinez-Lopez, D.G., Funderburg, N.T., Cerissi, A., Rifaie, R., *et al.* (2014) 'Lipopolysaccharide and soluble CD14 in cord blood plasma are associated with prematurity and chorioamnionitis.' *Pediatr. Res. 75*, 67–74.

Mead, M.N. (2008) 'Contaminants in human milk: Weighing the risks against the benefits of breastfeeding.' *Environ. Health Perspect. 116*, 10, A427–A434.

Mischke, M. and Plosch, T. (2013) 'More than just a gut instinct – the potential interplay between a baby's nutrition, its gut microbiome, and the epigenome.' *Am. J. Physiol. Regul. Integr. Comp. Physiol. 304*, R1065–R1069.

Neu, J. (2007) 'Perinatal and neonatal manipulation of the intestinal microbiome: A note of caution.' *Nutr. Rev. 65*, 282–285.

Neufeld, K.M., Kang, N., Bienenstock, J., and Foster, J.A. (2011) 'Reduced anxiety-like behavior and central neurochemical change in germ-free mice.' *Neurogastroenterol. Motil. 23*, 3, 255–264, e119.

Newburg, D.S. (2013) 'Glycobiology of human milk.' *Biokhimiya 78*, 7, 990–1007.

Nieuwdorp, M., Gilijamse, P.W., Pai, N., and Kaplan, L.M. (2014) 'Role of the microbiome in energy regulation and metabolism.' *Gastroenterology 146*, 1525–1533.

Palmer, C.N., Irvine, A.D., Terron-Kwiatkowski, A., Zhao, Y., *et al.* (2006) 'Common loss-of-function variants of the epidermal barrier protein filaggrin are a major predisposing factor for atopic dermatitis.' *Nat. Genet. 38*, 441–446.

Perez-Burgos, A., Wang, B., Mao, Y.K., Mistry, B., *et al.* (2013) 'Psychoactive bacteria *Lactobacillus rhamnosus* (JB-1) elicits rapid frequency facilitation in vagal afferents.' *Am. J. Physiol. Gastrointest. Liver Physiol. 304*, 2, G211–G220.

Porges, S. (2011) *The Polyvagal Theory: Neurophysiological Foundations of Emotions, Attachment, Communication, and Self-Regulation.* New York: Norton.

Putignani, L., Del Chierico, F., Petrucca, A., Vernocchi, P., and Dallapiccola, B. (2014) 'The human gut microbiota: A dynamic interplay with the host from birth to senescence settled during childhood.' *Pediatr. Res. 76*, 2–10.

Schultz, S.T., Klonoff-Cohen, H.S., Wingard, D.L., Akshoomoff, N.A., Macera, C.A., Ji, M. (2008) 'Acetaminophen (paracetamol) use, measles-mumps-rubella vaccination, and autistic disorder: the results of a parent survey.' *Autism, 12*, 3, 293–307.

Schultz S.T. and Gould G.G. (2016) 'Acetaminophen Use for Fever in Children Associated with Autism Spectrum Disorder.' *Autism Open Access, 6*, 2, 170.

Shaw, W. (2013) 'Evidence that increased acetaminophen use in genetically vulnerable children appears to be a major cause of the epidemics of autism, attention deficit with hyperactivity, and asthma.' *Journal of restorative medicine, 2*, 1–16.

Stiling, R.M., Dinan, T.J., and Cryan, J.F. (2014) 'Microbial genes, brain & behaviour – epigenetic regulation of the gut–brain axis.' *Genes, Brain and Behavior 13*, 1, 69–86.

Strachan, D.P. (1989) 'Hay fever, hygiene and household size.' *Br. Med. J. 299*, 1259–1260.

Sudo, N., Chida, Y., Aiba, Y., Sonoda, J., *et al.* (2004) 'Postnatal microbial colonization programs the hypothalamic-pituitary-adrenal system for stress response in mice.' *J. Physiol. 558 (Pt 1)*, 263–275.

Theije, C.G., Worperisis, H., and Ramadan, M. (2014) 'Altered gut microbiota and activity in a murine model of autism spectrum disorders.' *Brain Behav. Immun. 37*, 197–206.

Turroni, F., Ventura, M., Buttó, L.F., Duranti, S. *et al.* (2014) 'Molecular dialogue between the human gut microbiota and the host: A *Lactobacillus* and *Bifidobacterium* perspective.' *Cell Mol. Life Sci. 71*, 183–203.

Underwood, M.A., German, J.B., Lebrilla, C.B. and Mills, D.A. (2015) '*Bifidobacterium longum* subspecies *infantis*: Champion colonizer of the infant gut.' *Pediatr. Res. 77*, 229–235.

Weng, M. and Walker, W.A. (2013) 'The role of gut microbiota in programming the immune phenotype.' *J. Dev. Orig. Health Dis. 4*, 203–214.

CHAPTER 10

INTERVENTIONS AT BIRTH AND HOW TO WORK WITH THEM

John Wilks

Treating babies and children

This chapter outlines some of the issues relating to interventions at birth that may need addressing in sessions with babies and children. Approaches to treatment will vary depending on a therapist's expertise, but along with other applications outlined in this book it will usually involve physical touch or possibly work 'off the body' if touch is too activating. I would draw the reader's attention to some of the important considerations outlined in the introduction around creating a calm environment, working from the heart and always with permission.

A lot has been said already about the importance of creating a coherent, heart-based relational field within the clinic setting. Physical contact with babies, particularly around areas they have met with difficulty in the pregnancy or birth, needs to be negotiated very carefully. Remaining within a baby's 'window of tolerance' will ensure that a baby does not get overwhelmed or recapitulate held trauma. This is also true of parents; if they get overwhelmed by something in the session (guilt, shame or their own trauma) this will not create a safe contained space where babies can really let go and express what they need to. In these circumstances a baby may get the message that 'it is not safe for me to express what I need'. Gaining permission from a baby to make contact is not as straightforward as asking an adult (although it is essential for a therapist to also ask permission from the mum before they make any physical contact with her baby).

Babies will display clear body language about where they need touch and where they definitely do not want to be touched. However, making contact without proper negotiation can actually reinforce a trauma pattern in the body. Trying to 'fix' something physically when a baby is resisting you is certainly not helpful and usually makes symptoms worse. It can reinforce patterns such as 'I will never be listened to'. Respecting when babies push your hand away from an area you are attempting to make contact with can be an affirming gesture for babies when they realize they have control over the situation. They do not have to endure being compressed or stuck or having things done to them they don't want or are painful.

When we try to analyse the effects of certain experiences on babies, it is tempting to break them down into parts without looking at the baby as a whole. Therapists working with babies might be interested in the effects of their pre- and perinatal experience, but the fact is that all interventions will affect a baby's psychology, beliefs, immune system, cellular health, musculoskeletal system, autonomic nervous system and more – all at once. It's all very well treating a baby's tight diaphragm by using a particular physical technique for releasing it, but if we can hold a wider awareness about other factors related to why their diaphragm might have been tight in the first place, we are going to get a much better and deeper response.

For the baby, both pregnancy and birth are essentially sensory experiences which imprint the very tissues of their bodies as a 'felt sense'. This is why difficult early experience can be hard to rationalize later in life. This is the difference between 'implicit' and 'explicit' memory as outlined in Chapter 7. These implicit memories tend to get imprinted in our bodies and become so familiar that we don't realize that they are ruling how we interact and feel about the world and the people we are with. Our experiences shape our biology in the same way that our physical form is shaped by the movements and sensations of life in the womb.

When working with babies, we have to bear in mind that most healing happens in and through the body. A baby's felt sense of her own body can only change when that body is listened to, and allowed to resolve at its own pace and in its own way. As parents and therapists our ability to 'hear' and heal is predominantly limited by our belief system and, to a much lesser extent, our skill. In turn, our skill is dependent on how much we can use our subtler faculties, and trust our ability to 'tune in and listen'. By 'hearing' and 'listening' I mean using all our senses, not just our ears. Our hands become our sixth sense. We are listening to a life, and possibly even a pre-life, story as it is expressed in a body. Babies' bodies are highly sensitive and finely tuned and are much more sensitive to their external environment than we give them credit for.

A number of therapists will have undergone training to work physically with babies but this does not mean that their approaches are remotely the same. Some therapists will use a highly interventionist approach whilst others will be so cautious that the baby will not feel it has been 'met'. Somehow we need a happy medium where we are as engaged with a baby as we can, within our, its and its parents' windows of tolerance.

Ways of using physical touch within a therapy session are discussed here and in the following chapter. Having said that, this is not something that can really be learned from a book.

A baby's experience of birth

For a therapist, understanding what the experience of birth was like for a baby is vital. Many mums will relate that a birth was 'natural', 'normal', 'easy' or 'quick'. However, this does not mean by any stretch of the imagination that it was 'easy' or 'normal' for the baby. Particularly if the birth was quick, and therefore often 'easy' for the mum, it was almost certainly not easy or comfortable for the baby.

It is worth saying at this point that the terms 'natural birth' or 'normal birth' are used fairly casually but are not really accurate descriptions of what happens. One could hardly describe a baby's experience of birth as being a 'normal' experience! Even in an ideal situation it is intense on every level. Although it is important to get a full story from the parents about how the pregnancy and birth was for them, we also need to be aware that mothers (and fathers) can go into a dissociative state when talking about the birth, or they may have been so tired or drugged that they actually don't remember much of it. A mother who has had an epidural will have little idea about how difficult it might have been for her baby. However, a baby will remember everything, at least as a bodily 'felt sense', and display this clearly through their body language.

The desire to have a 'natural' birth can potentially set up feelings of disappointment in mums if things don't go to plan (which they rarely do), and this can disrupt mother–father–baby relationships. Fathers can feel that they didn't do enough to protect their partner, and mothers can feel they didn't do enough to protect their baby. It can be very helpful for therapists to be positive and relate from their own experience about how difficulties have actually enhanced their lives and how understanding, listening and compassion can go a long way to healing birth trauma. Even the term 'birth trauma' can evoke exaggerated ideas in mothers of lasting damage to their baby. Every mum wants the best for her baby, and guilt and disappointment are not happy bedfellows with early parenting. As Matthew Appleton has explained (see Chapter 5), trauma is much more to do with a baby's perception and what the relational field was like at the time rather than purely the mechanics of what happened. One baby's trauma is another's enriching experience. Reassurance that trauma can be healed and used as a positive experience is a vital element of all therapeutic approaches along with the expertise to know when to refer if a situation is outside our scope of practice or a baby needs urgent medical attention.

'Normal' vs 'natural'

It is important to understand that whereas 'natural' childbirth is usually defined as one where there is little or no human intervention, 'normal' birth may also include interventions to help the progress of labour, such as:

- augmentation of labour (by artificially stimulating contractions through the use of synthetic oxytocin)

- artificial rupture of the membranes

- pharmacologic pain relief (nitrous oxide, opioids and/or epidural)

- managed third stage of labour (this might include the use of Syntometrine or oxytocin to induce delivery of the placenta along with early cutting of the cord)

- non-pharmacologic pain relief (such as massage, hypnobirthing)

- intermittent foetal auscultation (listening to the baby's heart with a hand-held ultrasound or acoustical device such as a Sonicaid).

Within most national guidelines, a normal birth does not include things such as elective induction of labour prior to 41 weeks, forceps, ventouse,

Caesareans, routine episiotomy or continuous electronic foetal monitoring for low-risk birth.

Another consideration is that although many hospitals encourage skin-to-skin holding and breastfeeding in the first hour after birth, and mothers may report that they held their baby after birth, there may well have been some separation. Many mums and hospitals do not take into account the extreme importance of immediate and uninterrupted skin-to-skin contact after birth, or delayed cord clamping. It is interesting that practices such as augmentation of labour, early cord clamping and rupturing of the membranes are described as 'normal'. The sad fact is that a truly natural, undisturbed birth is very rare nowadays. It is therefore very important for therapists to ascertain exactly what happened at birth.

Babies and pain

The fact that some element of the birth might have been hard or painful or frightening for a baby is not something that necessarily occurs to parents. Culturally we still assume that babies won't remember painful experiences and it won't affect them. Certain practices such as foetal scalp monitoring and ventouse are extremely painful. As we will see, some of the effects such as inflammation, swelling and pain can persist for several weeks after birth and cause considerable discomfort for a baby, perhaps something analogous to having severe whiplash.

So, why do we continue to expose babies in the womb and newborns to such intensely painful experiences? A lot of assumptions around babies and pain are based on how a baby's brain develops. However, in terms of the longer-term effects of early exposure to pain, it is now thought that this can result in rewiring of the nerve pathways responsible for pain transmission, leading to increased sensation of pain (Page 2004). In other words, people who are exposed to early painful experiences become more sensitive to pain generally and are less able to tolerate it. Given the huge rise in incidence of chronic pain in our adult population, this connection needs to be considered seriously.

This has ramifications for common practices such as circumcision. Many therapists will be asked their opinion on circumcision. Around a third of all males in the world are circumcised, mostly without any form of anaesthesia.

This usually happens around 10 days after birth but can be anywhere between a week and adolescence.

The *Surgical Guide to Circumcision* (Bolnick, Koyle and Yosha 2012) states that: 'all of the nerve pathways essential for the transmission and perception of pain are present and functioning by 24 weeks' gestation... If untreated, the pain of circumcision can cause both short- and long-term changes in infant behavior.' Despite this, circumcision is still advocated by some books on baby care.

For the sake of convenience, the rest of this chapter is divided into two parts; first, information that will help practitioners understand the dynamics of working with babies who have been exposed to pharmacological interventions; and second, with babies who have had mechanical interventions such as Caesarean, forceps or suction.

PART 1: PHARMACOLOGICAL INFLUENCES

The unsettled baby – not just the birth?

There may be a myriad of reasons why a baby is unsettled. Fast or difficult births (at least from the baby's perspective) may be one reason, but there are numerous other potential factors that might have arisen during the pregnancy as well. Some of these have been discussed earlier in terms of maternal stress, family dynamics, attempted termination or even whether a baby was planned or wanted. Other factors might be related to the use of recreational or medicinal drugs during pregnancy, pain-relieving drugs at birth, or antibiotics. One of the often overlooked reasons for a distressed baby is the maternal use of antidepressants during pregnancy, so it is essential for practitioners to ask what medications, if any, were taken during this time.

Antidepressants

The use of the SSRI group of antidepressants during pregnancy is highly controversial. Pregnant women are bombarded with cautionary advice about not exposing their unborn baby to even small amounts of substances such as alcohol, but when it comes to pharmaceuticals there is little clear information available, with drugs often being assumed safe in pregnancy unless proved otherwise. The difficulty that a mother who is on antidepressant medication faces when discovering that she is pregnant cannot be overemphasized, and getting good medical advice is vital. The SSRI group consists of drugs such as Fluoxetine (Prozac, Prizma, Flutine, Affectine), Paroxetine[1] (Seroxat, Paxxet, Paxil), Sertraline (Lustral, Zoloft), Fluvoxamine (Favoxil, Luvox), Citalopram (Cipramil, Recital), Escitalopram (Ciprodex, Cipralex) and Venlafaxine (Effexor, Venla, Viepax).

Long-term consequences of SSRI use during pregnancy

The effect on the foetus of being subjected to extremely high doses of antidepressants whilst in the womb is something that has not been researched well. Side-effects in adults can include such unpleasant symptoms as agitation, dizziness and anxiety. It has also been found that, like adults, babies can suffer after birth from 'discontinuation syndrome', the equivalent of cold turkey, similar to what is seen with babies born of narcotic addicts. Up to a third of these babies will be jittery and inconsolable, have tremors and diarrhoea, and display respiratory distress, which may resolve within three to five days but can last up to one month.

It is very difficult to say how SSRIs might affect a developing baby. Because embryological development is so incredibly complex and involves the simultaneous and interrelated development of many different systems at once (gastrointestinal, nervous, musculoskeletal, etc.), and is dependent on the complex and finely balanced array of circulating hormones and neurotransmitters, it would probably be safe to say, not particularly well. It is known that serotonin plays a key role in the development of the foetal brain as well as the regulation of appetite, mood, temperature and the perception of pain. Animal studies have shown that exposure to SSRIs at certain vulnerable embryonic stages can induce changes in foetal brain circulation resulting in long-lasting behavioural effects.

Various names have been given to symptoms of withdrawal that babies suffer from, including neonatal abstinence syndrome (NAS), which is seen in about 30 per cent of all babies exposed to SSRIs, the main symptoms

---

1   Paroxetine is also known as Brisdelle, which has been licensed for hot flushes linked to menopause in the USA and comes with a pregnancy category X warning.

being hypoactivity, lethargy, a weak cry and hypotonia. These symptoms then rapidly change to jitteriness, poor feeding, irritability, respiratory distress and abnormal crying. The long-term effects have not been evaluated. Breastfeeding has been shown to decrease the severity of NAS, which is not surprising given its calming effect on babies, but again, studies of the long-term effects on breast-fed infants are lacking. Therapies that have a similar calming effect on babies such as baby massage, craniosacral and Bowen work would appear to be most useful in this situation.

Induction and augmentation

Induction or augmentation of labour usually involves the use of prostaglandins (in the form of a pessary) or intravenous oxytocin (Pitocin or Syntocinon). All births can be fast, but induction tends to have specific consequences. Babies who are born fast or who have been induced are often difficult to settle. For therapists, their nervous systems can often feel 'jangled' or 'wired' in a state of sympathetic arousal.

So what does it feel like to be induced? Without wanting to sound overdramatic, the experience for the baby is probably similar to the sensation of drowning. The birth activist Doris Haire described the effects of induction on the baby as 'analogous to holding an infant under the surface of the water, allowing the infant to come to the surface to gasp for air, but not to breathe' (Buckley 2009). The type of body language the babies might display in this situation is discussed in Chapter 6. Induction also means that 'conjunct sites', where the baby comes up against hard and bony areas of the mum's pelvis, might well hold more charge for a baby as the forces involved are harder, faster, less controlled and painful. These places (usually areas of the cranium) will often show up in baby body language; the baby may touch them repeatedly but will need careful negotiation around any therapeutic touch in these areas.

From the mum's point of view, induction inhibits the body's own production of endorphins, her natural painkillers, leading to increased need for epidurals and other pain-killing medication. For the baby, such a birth, particularly if pain-relieving drugs are used, can result in the imprinting that sleep and 'letting go' is somehow dangerous and they have to fight it at all costs. They have to remain hypervigilant. Sometimes these babies will wake up suddenly and display the Moro reflex (the baby startle reflex) as they begin to drop off to sleep. Clients and friends who have had children who have been induced relate that tendencies from this kind of birth persist into teenage years and adulthood, with them being highly resistant to getting ready to go out, or getting them out of the house ready for school in the morning.

Oxytocin – natural or synthetic?

Synthetic oxytocin has a very different effect to the finely balanced hormonal cascade that is released during birth. Oxytocin is just part of a cocktail of hormones that stimulate bonding for both baby and mother. Oxytocin is often described as the hormone of love whilst beta-endorphins encourage dependency, and prolactin produces the mothering instinct. They all work together with vasopressin in a complex cocktail to encourage positive bonding behaviours.

Pitocin and Syntocinon are chemically identical to oxytocin, but because of the blood–brain barrier, it affects the brain and central nervous system differently. Mothers do not get the relaxing, anti-anxiety benefit of the cascade of hormones or the feelings of love and containment that naturally produced oxytocin gives. The baby also produces its own oxytocin, which no doubt helps it deal with the rigours of being born and imprints an association of love and bonding on an otherwise difficult experience. Specifically, what happens is that oxytocin affects the baby's brain chemistry in a way that calms it during delivery and makes it less prone to damage resulting from lack of oxygen.

Long-term effects of induction

The link between oxytocin exposure and later behaviour is a complex one, but it is known that disruption of normal oxytocin mechanisms plays a role in antisocial behaviour and aggression. Professor Sue Carter of the Department of Psychiatry at the University of Illinois at Chicago has studied prairie voles as they have similar bonding behaviours to humans. Her research found that whereas low doses of oxytocin facilitated later social behaviour, high doses (such as are used in induction) disrupted pair bond formation as adults (Carter *et al.* 2009). By interfering in such a complex process as birth we may be playing a dangerous game of roulette with the psychological and physical health of our offspring.

Endogenous oxytocin (i.e. produced by the mother) also has some other less well-known advantages. As it is produced during breastfeeding, it lowers the stress response and encourages bonding. Oxytocin seems to be involved in prompting maternal behaviour rather than maintaining it, so a mother's exposure to oxytocin at the time of birth would appear to be crucial. Interestingly, oxytocin is higher in mothers who interact for the first time with young children who are not their own rather than their own children, proving its crucial role in initial bonding behaviour. Other concerns that are known about the synthetic use of oxytocin include the fact that breastfeeding may be more difficult as a result of breast engorgement (which makes it more difficult for the baby to latch on) and it can also lead to the desensitization of breast tissue (Lewis 2012).

The effect of pain-relieving drugs

In terms of pain relief there are a number of different drugs that are used, and although we don't know exactly the specific effects on the baby, we do know some of the short and long-term ramifications on things such as feeding, bonding and brain development. Concerns about pain relief have been expressed since the 1970s but, if anything, its use in childbirth has become more widespread and there is still hardly any research looking at longer-term consequences for the child.

Pethidine

Because pethidine remains in the newborn's bloodstream for at least 62 hours it can cause irritability and feeding problems. It is therefore important to ascertain whether such drugs were used. Pethidine is found in breast milk, so that a baby will continue to receive the drug for the next few days after birth. Even after seven days, the after-effects of pethidine can cause babies to be less alert, harder to settle and to cry more easily when disturbed. Pethidine can create a 'fogginess' in the baby during the crucial 24-hour period after birth and affect bonding.

There are longer-term effects of pethidine as well. Women remember their birth experiences vividly for the rest of their lives. The sedative effect of pethidine may affect recall, impacting negatively on what is one of the most important events in a mother's life. It is known that babies exposed to pethidine are more likely to cry when handled and are less able to settle, something that is seen up to six weeks after birth, although the longer-term effects have not been studied.

Narcotics cross the placenta and depress the central nervous system, with the potential to affect breathing in the newborn baby. If there is a maternal drop in blood pressure, there can be a reduced blood flow in the placenta, which might show up as umbilical baby body language during therapy.

Epidurals and spinal analgesia

In an epidural, a local anaesthetic is injected into the space beneath the dura mater. When an epidural is administered, the body thinks that there is no pain and levels of beta-endorphins drop very dramatically. At the time of birth, a woman with an epidural has about 20 per cent of the beta-endorphin levels of a woman after a normal birth.

For the baby, some of the ramifications of epidurals may include:

- Foetal distress as a result of lowered maternal blood pressure.

- Greater likelihood that labour will be augmented.

- Less chance that a baby will turn from a posterior position, making a posterior, and therefore more painful, birth more likely. Babies who are born this way will often display compression at the base of the occiput as a lot of pressure is exerted here as the baby is pushed hard against the top of the mum's sacrum.

- Increased likelihood of instrumental deliveries (forceps and ventouse). It has also been shown that where epidurals and forceps are used, around twice as much force is applied to the baby than would happen if the mother was not medicated. This is very important from the baby's point of view.

- Epidural drugs pass through to the baby and take longer for them to eliminate than an adult. Residues have been found in the newborn's urine 36 hours after birth.

- Babies born after epidurals seem to be less alert, less able to orient, and have less mature motor function even a month after birth.

Pharmacological interventions after birth: antibiotics

Antibiotics are given routinely to both mothers and babies, typically in the following situations:

- where a mother has Group B strep (GBS); GBS is bacterial and is normally treated with intravenous antibiotics during labour or given to the baby after birth

- in severe maternal infection such as meningitis or pneumonia

- as a preventive measure in Caesarean sections

- following prolonged rupture of the membranes (usually in excess of 24 hours)

- with some premature babies.

Some antibiotics should not be used in pregnancy at all, specifically tetracyclines (minocycline, doxycycline) and fluoroquinolones (ciprofloxacin, levofloxacin, moxifloxacin), as well as sulfasalazine and nitrofurantoin (for urine infections).

All uses will have an effect on the baby's microbiome, particularly as it would appear that the gut and the immune system are effectively 'primed' at birth through contact with the flora in the vagina, through skin-to-skin contact and breastfeeding. It is known, for example, that babies who are given antibiotics before they are one year old have around a 40 per cent increased chance of developing eczema, with each additional course increasing the risk by 7 per cent (Tsakok *et al.* 2013).

Babies may be exposed to antibiotics through breastfeeding or by being given antibiotics directly. The most common broad-spectrum antibiotics that are used are penicillin (ampicillin or amoxicillin) or sometimes erythromycin. Advice from the manufacturers of these drugs alerts the user to the fact that they may cause diarrhoea and rashes in the breast-fed infant as a result of sensitization, or, in the case of ampicillin, that there may be an increase in cases of diarrhoea and thrush (candidiasis) attributed to ampicillin in breast milk. A recent study has also shown a link between early antibiotic use and the development of obesity in children (Ajslev *et al.* 2011).

Along with pharmacological drugs there may also have been mechanical interventions at birth which have their own consequences and require specific approaches to treatment.

PART 2: PHYSICAL IMPRINTING AT BIRTH – MECHANICAL INTERVENTIONS

Although birth itself exerts huge forces on the baby, there are other physical pressures that occur during pregnancy as well. We are shaped by our position or 'birth lie' in the womb, whether that is anterior, posterior (back-to-back), side-lying, breech or caught up under the ribs. Most positions involve a degree of lengthening through one side of the body and this will manifest later in life in characteristics such as a slightly lower eye on one side, and a corresponding asymmetry in the pelvis and leg-length discrepancy.

Compression forces seem to be important in nature in terms of biological formation. Like most other creatures, we are born through a narrow space, which involves being squeezed. Cranial osteopaths talk about this process of compression and expansion as one of instigating 'ignition' in the cerebrospinal fluid and in the baby's system generally. For the baby, the sense of compression gets more and more intense during the last trimester as it has less and less room to move around. During birth itself, these compressive forces can feel extreme, initially as the baby's head comes up against the cervix and then as it negotiates its way down the birth canal.

Because of the size of the baby's head and the shape of the mum's pelvis, humans are unique in that rotation has to occur in order for the baby to be born. Because of our large brain size, we are born effectively nine months early in relation to other developmental factors. This is why the whole notion of babies being born into an 'external womb environment' is so crucial for therapists to understand. Most other mammals are able to function much more independently right after birth, being able to walk, see, hear and interact within a few days.

The other kind of strong mechanical force that is unique to humans is traction. As discussed shortly, this is an unusual force from a physiological point of view as a baby's body is not naturally designed for it. Strong compressive forces are par for the course in almost every kind of birth in every species. But traction is something that is distinctly human unless you happen to be a calf or sheep that was stuck and dragged out by a farmer. Traction is applied in various ways during human births; at Caesareans, through the use of forceps or ventouse and even in 'normal' births. Some of these can be reasonably gentle whilst others require all the strength of an obstetrician.

Rotational forces experienced during birth

Rotation as the baby comes down the birth canal causes dragging and torsion in the various articulations of the baby's cranium and the neck. Many of these patterns can be held in the softer bones such as the parietals or the squama of the occiput. However, for therapists it is important to address patterns that are held in the harder, more cartilaginous base of the cranium such as the base of the occiput, the sphenoid and the petrous portion of the temporal bones.

Osteopaths and chiropractors have observed that the majority of us have a degree of imbalance at the occipito-atlantal joint resulting from rotational patterns experienced at birth. Rotational forces also affect the jaw and the TMJ. In the opinion of many health professionals, these imbalances can lead to distortions elsewhere in the body; specifically, they have a marked effect on posture, with a more general knock-on effect on efficient functioning. This is not surprising because, as we will see, many important fascial connections descend from the cranial base. Dr Niall Galloway (Galloway 2016) has pointed out that small imbalances towards the top of the body get amplified further down the body; small torsion or rotational patterns at the occipito-atlantal joint will show up as obvious distortions in the pelvis. Indeed, some paediatric dentists work extensively with the relationship between posture and bite, improving spinal curvature by adjusting a child's bite (Levinkind 2008). Forces of compression and rotation can be more pronounced with posterior births, common with first-time mothers, which either leads to a longer rotation or, in some cases, interventions such as epidurals or Caesareans.

Treatment approaches

Every baby could benefit from some treatment after birth, and in a few hospitals cranial osteopathy or craniosacral therapy is offered routinely to babies who have been through a difficult birth. Many inter-osseous and intra-osseous patterns are much easier to rectify if addressed early, although this is not to say that healing cannot occur at any stage of life. On a physical level, the kind of physical issues that therapists encounter with babies include:

- compression, torsion, rotation and traction (e.g. between vertebrae or the bones of the skull)

- micro-tearing of the tissues (through interventions such as suction, forceps or Caesarean section)

- inflammation (through over-stretching of the tissues or as a result of a surgical intervention)

- nerve compression (e.g. the nerve that supplies some of the muscles in the neck or some of the cranial nerves that affect eye movement)

- stretching of a nerve or nerve root such as might happen in a brachial plexus injury (neurapraxia, or neuroma)

- blood supply to tissues or organs, which might be compromised by restrictions in the fascia

- nasal and oral issues (e.g. blocked tear ducts or an unusually high or low palate)

- muscle tension (e.g. through the diaphragm, neck or psoas muscles, exhibiting a protective pattern)

- patterns within the bones themselves (termed intra-osseous patterns).

Therapeutically it is more beneficial to work on babies and children as soon as possible (bearing in mind that it is best to avoid any disruption during the first week of life) to avoid patterns being set up that might be more difficult to rectify later in life. Many of the moulding patterns that are obviously visible to a mother are not necessarily the most important to address. Part of the reason for this is that the cranial vault, which is quite membranous in an infant, is the most visible part of the infant skull and most prone to moulding, whereas the cranial base is denser. The cranial base is important to address from a structural point of view because of the fascial connections that arise here and form strong relationships with the whole of the rest of the body (described below).

Part of the reason why it is so much easier to work on infants and babies is that whereas some parts of the skull begin to ossify by week 11 and are fully formed at birth, other parts don't completely fuse until about 12 years old. For example, the mastoid portions of the temporal bones ossify during the second year after birth and the sacrum sometimes not until late teens. It is easy to see torsion patterns that had their origin in birth when examining adult craniums and sacrums; the patterns become ossified in distinct shapes that tell the story of their birth.

What structures are affected by birth?

Some therapists will work with specific structures according to their expertise, but really babies' bones, membranes, fascia, sinuses and nervous system are inextricably intertwined. You can't treat one without having an effect on all the others.

Cranial bones

The cranial bones develop very early in the foetus from the mesenchymal tissue at the end of the notochord, where a condensation of cells begins to happen around the end of week four. Most of the cranial base derives from cartilage, and the base of the occiput at the foramen magnum becomes cartilaginous around week five or six. The ethmoid bone (which forms the anterior attachment of the falx) begins to ossify by week 11 and is fully ossified at birth, but parts of the sphenoid are formed from membrane and don't fully ossify until about 12 years old.

Fascial connections

There are good reasons why forces exerted on the head will be transmitted further down the body and create potential postural issues. Most of this 'force transmission' happens through the bands and tubes of fascia that hang off various areas of the base of the cranium as well as the core connection that osteopaths talk about, which is the meningeal fascia that surrounds the brain and spinal cord. This tube (the dura mater, and to a certain degree the arachnoid and pia membranes) attaches to the sacrum, the top of the neck and the base of the cranium and creates a very strong reciprocal relationship between the head, neck and lower back.

Some of the main fascial connections that arise from the base of the cranium include the following:

- The *investing fascia* arises from the occipital protuberance and superior nuchal crest, the zygomatic arch, masseter, mandible and hyoid. It thickens at various places to form structures such as the stylomandibular ligament.

- The *pretracheal fascia* descends from the mandible and hyoid and covers the anterior and posterior aspects of the trachea. It connects with the thyroid via Berry's ligament (which is a suspensory ligament). Important thickening occurs around the apex of each lung (the suprapleural membrane or Sibson's fascia) so that issues here can affect lymphatic drainage.

- The *carotid sheaths* (which are very tough) lie posterior to the pretracheal fascia and are connected medially by the alar fascia which in turn merges anteriorly and inferiorly with the buccopharyngeal fascia and the pericardium. The carotid sheaths are also connected loosely with the prevertebral fascia which forms a tube around the cervical vertebrae and the deep cervical muscles. Inferiorly it is continuous with the longitudinal ligaments of the vertebral column. The anterior tube is continuous with the pericardium and diaphragm.

- The *buccopharyngeal fascia* descends from the cranial base and pterygoid processes of the sphenoid to enclose the trachea and oesophagus. It is continuous with the pretracheal fascia and merges with the pericardium of the heart.

- The *alar fascia* merges with the buccopharyngeal fascia and pericardium. The prevertebral fascia is continuous with the connective tissue of the vertebral column down to the sacrum. Prevertebral fascia also has some connections posteriorly to the trapezius and anteriorly to the anterior longitudinal ligament of T1, T2 and T3.

- From the diaphragm there is a continuity of fascia via the crura to the psoas, the falciform ligament of the liver, the round ligament and the umbilical ligament down to the pubic arch and posteriorly to the sacrum.

When you bear in mind these intricate connections it is easy to understand why tensional forces anywhere in the body will reflect everywhere else and why imbalances at the cranial base can have such profound ramifications elsewhere in the body. To really understand these connections, I would draw the reader's attention to the pioneers of the concept and practical application of biotensegrity, including Dr Stephen Levin, Tom Flemons, Donald Ingber, Danielle-Claude Martin, Graham Scarr, Tom Myers, John Sharkey and Joanne Avison.

The shoulder and brachial plexus

As the baby emerges, the posterior shoulder is naturally born first, with the anterior (normally the right) shoulder having to negotiate under the mother's pubic arch. This can exert strain on the shoulder and nerves supplying the arm. For some reason, some obstetricians will birth the anterior shoulder first, which can put excessive strain on this area and can lead to brachial plexus injuries (BPIs), particularly if the mother is trying to give birth lying on her back.

At birth, injuries can be caused by shoulder dystocia (SD), where the shoulder becomes stuck under the pubic arch. This can happen if a baby is very large or very overdue but is more often due to factors such as epidurals where mothers have a lack of sensation, obstetric intervention and particularly induction. One of the key aids to prevent this is the position of the mother during birth, as lying on one's back significantly decreases the space front to back in the pelvis. BPIs are sometimes referred to by different names (brachial plexus palsy, Horner's syndrome or torticollis).

One of the most sensitive areas of the cranium prone to compressive forces are the temporal bones. There are a lot of structures around them which are vulnerable to both compression and also to traction forces used in some births. There are many types of birth that put excessive strain on this area, notably forceps (strong compressive and rotational forces) and ventouse (traction and rotational forces).

As discussed shortly, traction has specific consequences for a baby's body and nervous system. Pulling on the head or neck will feel threatening, and a baby will do all it can to protect itself by contracting the sub-occipital and deep abdominal muscles such as the psoas, resulting in the commonly seen response of bringing the knees up towards the chest. This is part of an instinctive reflex to protect the vulnerable areas of its body, particularly the abdomen and the brainstem. These reflex tendencies can persist after birth, resulting in symptoms such as colic, and perhaps even into adulthood manifesting as symptoms such as back pain.

Tissue memory from birth

One of the fascinating things when working therapeutically is that it is not uncommon for a therapist to sense very specific incidents where a particular birth trauma might have occurred. Sometimes whilst working with an adult, the cranium under your hands can feel very small as though you are holding an infant's skull, or their whole body might express a pattern directly linked to birth. In craniosacral work, no force is used to encourage the body to release these patterns. By 'listening' through your hands the 'Blueprint energy' that David Haas talked about in Chapter 7 is allowed to express itself through the tissues and the body will 'unwind' and let go of these patterns. In cranial osteopathy this is sometimes referred to as allowing the potency in the tissues to express itself. For craniosacral therapists the starting point is always paying attention to the various rhythms and 'tides' of the body as they are expressed through the tissues. These tide-like rhythms are described briefly in the section on craniosacral therapy in Chapter 12.

It is said that 'what the mind forgets, the body remembers', but often when the adult body is allowed to remember through therapy, the mind remembers it too and the conceptual understanding that happens through this process can be immensely healing.

Plagiocephaly and brachycephaly

'Flat head syndrome' has become much more prevalent since 1994 when many national health organizations started advising parents that babies should sleep on their back rather than their front in order to lessen the chance of cot death or Sudden Infant Death Syndrome (SIDS). This has halved the incidence of SIDS but has had some inadvertent consequences, one of which is that babies develop less strength and co-ordination in their upper bodies than they used to, and can be slower to crawl. As a result, a common posture seen in children is anteriorly rotated shoulders and tight pectoral muscles which affects, amongst other things, the thoracic inlet, the brachial plexus and breathing patterns. The other consequence is a flattening of the back of the head, either on one side (plagiocephaly) or both sides (brachycephaly).

Fast births

We have looked at the ramifications of fast births on the microbiome and the 'seeding' of the gut flora that happens as the baby comes down the birth canal. In fast births this can be compromised. But more than that, the nervous systems of babies tend to work fairly slowly and they need time to adjust and 'catch their breaths' during the tortuous journey down the birth canal. They come up against numerous hard and unforgiving areas in the mum's pelvis and sacrum and will do a process of 'turtling' (so called because it resembles the way a turtle sticks its head out and retracts as it comes into contact with something external) as they negotiate the twists and turns of coming down the birth canal. Fast births tend to exacerbate the roughness of contact with parts of the mum's pelvis such as the top of the sacrum or the ischial spines. These areas are called 'conjunct' sites in the PPN literature and will often be areas that need attention from the therapist as they can hold various patterns such as compression, torsion, inflammation and, of course, pain. They will often be areas that are sensitive to touch and that a baby will repeatedly make contact with herself to demonstrate that attention is needed here.

Traction – forceps, suction, vacuum extraction and ventouse

Ventouse and forceps are extremely painful for a baby. It is a case where reparation by therapists and parents openly acknowledging the pain that a baby has been through can be a catalyst for healing. Such a birth can imprint on a baby such life statements as 'the world is a violent and painful place' or 'human touch is unsafe, painful, abrupt and uncaring'. It is not surprising that babies born this way can have a difficult time.

The use of forceps in births is less common these days in the USA, but they are still used in nearly 7 per cent of all births in the UK; whereas ventouse (or vacuum extraction as it is called in the USA) only came into mainstream use in the 1970s, with about 6 per cent of all births in the UK currently being assisted with suction caps. Apart from the strong traction on the neck, forceps also impact on certain cranial nerves such as the vagus, glossopharangeal and spinal accessory nerves. This might cause problems with digestion (e.g. colic or a sluggish digestive tract), hypertonus in the neck muscles, neck restriction (torticollis or wry neck is quite common) or feeding problems.

Suction puts an extremely strong local pressure on the squama of the occiput as well as pulling up the base of the cranium, particularly around the foramen magnum which is a strong attachment site for the dura. Ventouse exerts an extraordinary amount of force, which has the potential for distortion patterns to be fed into the baby's cranium, affecting such structures as the brain stem, venous sinuses and the TMJ. Most babies will be born with a chignon or caput, which is a dark circular swelling on the head, and sometimes blisters or larger abrasions. Babies can also get a cephalhaematoma, which is a collection of blood under the scalp next to the periosteum.

Practitioners can get a sense of distortion patterns around the cranial base by gently palpating the base of the occiput where it articulates with the atlas. Patterns might be felt as one side around the condyles being anterior or superior. It is easy to assess the temporal area by looking down from the top of the baby's head. If you look at the position of the ears you may notice that one is anterior to the other, or the TMJ is superior on one side. Work such as Bowen or craniosacral therapy can go a long way to rectifying these patterns.

Neck restrictions are also easy to observe as babies will often have their head to one side rather than the other when lying down, or prefer to feed from one breast rather than the other. It is also possible to test by getting the baby to follow the movement of your finger. Babies are naturally inquisitive and will follow any movement with their gaze and may resist following your movement.

Neck restrictions can also affect blood flow to the cranium, a pulling up of the brain stem, as well as stress on the short sub-occipital muscles, dural membranes, venous sinuses and ventricles (particularly the fourth ventricle) (Flanagan 2010). The vertebral artery, which supplies some of the blood to the brain, passes through foramina in the cervical vertebrae and then does a loop around the base of the occiput before entering the cranium. A restriction in blood supply would result from a neck restriction on either side.

A baby's occiput at birth is shown in Figure 10.1.

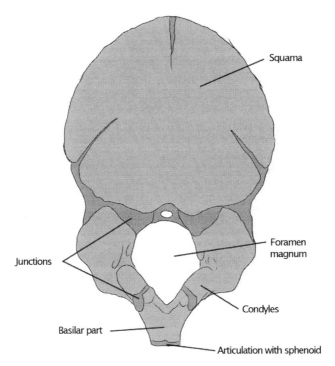

Figure 10.1 A baby's occiput at birth showing the junctions around the condyles and cranial base

The effect of traction on the psoas

The psoas muscles function as an important stabilizer of the back in the adult. They are particularly responsive to emotional states and have a tendency to contract if a baby feels unsafe. There is a strong reciprocal protective relationship between the psoas and the neck; when the psoas is tight the sub-occipitals tend to be tight and vice versa. The psoas can be affected if the umbilical cord is cut or clamped too soon, particularly before it has stopped pulsating. This premature cutting of the cord can be a severe shock for the newborn baby as the heart, liver and bladder undergo rapid transition to lung breathing. A remnant of our umbilical vein forms the falciform ligament that passes through our liver, and it is common for umbilical shock to be fed into that area. This will often show itself as specific baby body language in sessions.

The mouth and jaw

One of the major influences on the development of the hard palate and jaw is breastfeeding. The hard palate in a newborn has the consistency of soft wax, so it is very malleable. Research has generally shown that bottle-feeding results in more malocclusions as well as affecting the muscles involved in opening and closing the mouth (Labbok and Hendershot 1986). As opposed to an artificial teat or dummy, a woman's nipple expands in three directions – side to side, top to bottom and front to back – so that a baby's sucking action helps mould the internal space of the mouth and hence will determine bite and dentition later on.

Caesareans

There is a generally held perception that a Caesarean birth is the least stressful way to give birth for both mum and baby, but unfortunately this is far from true. Apart from frequent problems with bonding, babies born this way tend to have more respiratory and breathing difficulties and are more at risk of asthma, and conditions such as coeliac disease (Neu and Rushing 2011).

C-sections usually have to be performed quickly, though nowadays there is a move towards more 'natural' and slower Caesareans. Caesareans often involve strong traction and rotation of the baby's neck and immediate cord clamping. These forces strain the sensitive sub-occipital fascia, so it can be very beneficial for a baby to receive some craniosacral or Bowen treatment in the weeks after birth.

References

Ajslev, T.A., Andersen, C.S., Gamborg, M., Sørensen, T.I.A., and Jess, T. (2011) 'Childhood overweight after establishment of the gut microbiota: The role of delivery mode, pre-pregnancy weight and early administration of antibiotics.' *International Journal of Obesity 35*, 4, 522–529.

Bolnick, D.A., Koyle, M.A., and Yosha, A. (eds) (2012) *Surgical Guide to Circumcision.* London: Springer.

Buckley, S.J. (2009) 'Undisturbed Birth: Mother Nature's Blueprint for Safety, Ease and Ecstasy.' In *Gentle Birth, Gentle Mothering: The Wisdom and Science of Gentle Choices in Pregnancy, Birth, and Parenting.* Available at http://sarahbuckley.com/gentle-birth-gentle-mothering, accessed on 10 October 2016.

Carter, C.S., Boone, E., Grippo, A.J., Ruscio, M., and Bales, K.L. (2009) 'The Endocrinology of Social Relationships in Rodents.' In P.T. Ellison and P.B. Gray (eds) *Endocrinology of Social Relationships.* Cambridge, MA: Harvard University Press.

Flanagan, M. (2010) *The Downside of Upright Posture.* Minneapolis, MN: Two Harbors Press.

Galloway, N. (2016) *Pelvic Support Anatomy: A Biotensegrity Perspective.* Presentation at the British Fascia Symposium, Worcester, UK, 24 June 2016.

Labbok, M.H. and Hendershot, G.E. (1986) 'Does breastfeeding protect against malocclusion? An analysis of the 1981 Child Health Supplement to the National Health Interview Survey.' *American Journal of Preventive Medicine 3*, 4, 227–232.

Levinkind, M. (2008) *Consideration of Whole Body Posture in Relation to Dental Development and Treatment of Malocclusion in Children.* Available at www.drlevinkind.com/images/uploads/publication_ consideration-of-whole-body-posture%20v1.0.pdf, accessed on 10 October 2016.

Lewis, M.J. (2012) *An Investigation of the Effects of Pitocin for Labor Induction and Augmentation on Breastfeeding Success.* Available at http://scholarship.claremont.edu/cgi/viewcontent. cgi?article=1112&context=scripps_theses, accessed on 10 October 2016.

Neu, J. and Rushing, J. (2011) 'Cesarean versus vaginal delivery: Long-term infant outcomes and the hygiene hypothesis.' *Clinics in Perinatology 38*, 2, 321–331.

Page, G.G. (2004) 'Are there long-term consequences of pain in newborn or very young infants?' *The Journal of Perinatal Education 13*, 3, 10–17.

Tsakok, T., McKeever, T.M., Yeo, L., and Flohr, C. (2013) 'Does early life exposure to antibiotics increase the risk of eczema? A systematic review.' *British Journal of Dermatology 169*, 5, 983–991.

CHAPTER 11

EMOTIONAL FIRST AID FOR BABIES AND THEIR PARENTS

FUNDAMENTALS AND PRACTICE OF ATTACHMENT-BASED PARENT–INFANT BODY PSYCHOTHERAPY

Thomas Harms

Introduction

If we saw a house on fire, it would not make much sense to take time to study the history of its construction or the layout of its rooms. We wouldn't be interested in how the inhabitants relate to each other or what kinds of conflicts have not been resolved within the family. All this can wait, as the priority is to save everyone in the house who is in danger.

During a postnatal crisis, the house is, figuratively speaking, on fire. Instead of there being harmony within the household, a dangerous dynamic develops in which stress and growing insecurity cause the parents to lose their emotional bond with their infant. In recent literature, these insidious vicious cycles have been clearly described (Diederichs and Jungclaussen 2009; Harms 2008; Papousek, Schieche and Wurmser 2004). Due to the enormous amount of stress during such crises, the parents' empathic and intuitive abilities are increasingly undermined. For the infant, the rupture of the parental bond represents a dangerous situation if it persists for any length of time. The baby loses his sense of security and a safe haven in the world. Nowadays we know that brief losses of contact are a normal part of the interaction between a child and its parents, and under normal circumstances the infant has the ability to actively invite his primary caregivers to pick up the emotional thread again.

Lasting psychosocial burdens or unresolved traumatic stress from pregnancy, birth and the postnatal period can be fertile ground for this dynamic of tension, inability to relate, and estrangement. During these times, orientation gets lost, the ability to regulate emotions is no longer present, and even the parents' own baby can be perceived as threatening and rejecting. The infant responds to the loss of relational security with sustained increased muscle tone and by refusing touch and eye contact. Hectic, uncoordinated movements, increased whining and excessive crying are further symptoms indicating the acute loss of psycho-physical alignment between parents and their infant.

When parents have their backs to the wall like this, they can be overcome with impulses and fantasies to use violence against their baby. Therefore, efficient tools are urgently needed for them to regain stability and inner security. Emotional First Aid (EFA) is a systematic approach within modern body psychotherapy, specifically developed to accompany and overcome ruptures in the relationship between parents and their infant.

History and scientific influences of Emotional First Aid

The historic roots of EFA go back to the pioneering work of the physician, psychoanalyst and natural scientist Wilhelm Reich (1897–1957). In the 1940s, Reich developed his theories about how to apply his methods of body-oriented psychotherapy, which he called vegeto-therapy or orgone therapy, in short-term therapy with highly stressed parents, infants and young children (Reich 2010). It is in this context that Reich first mentions EFA (Reich 1987). His daughter Eva Reich, who worked as a physician and perinatologist in the USA, took up her father's preventive work, developed his methods further and made them into an important element of the preventive use of body psychotherapy which she called 'gentle bioenergetics' (Overly 2005; Reich and Zornànszky 1993).

In the mid-1980s Eva Reich started to visit Berlin on a regular basis where she taught her method of neurosis prevention and infant therapy in seminars (Meyer 2015). It was in that context that I first got to know about these body-based bioenergetic concepts of infant therapy. At the same time, I was following the then growing research into infant psychology and attachment, more specifically the newly discovered phenomenon of excessively crying babies. In the early 1990s I launched the first 'Crying Emergency Service' in the neighborhood center of the UFA factory in Berlin Tempelhof where parents with inconsolably crying babies could get help.

However, in the attempt to support and assist parents and their infants to get through the crisis, it soon became apparent that the currently developed tools were insufficient for the demands of crisis management. Massages, touch and expression techniques of Reichian therapy could only be applied in a very limited way. For instance, babies who had only little ability to soothe themselves would refuse the touch or cry even more which, in turn, would exacerbate their parents' distress.

These early experiences increasingly shifted the focus of our work towards a different direction. Instead of trying to loosen blockages in the emotional and physical expression of the child, other questions became central: What can be done, with the help of body psychotherapy, to strengthen the parents' intuitive relational abilities? How can approaches of body psychotherapy be used in order to give parents insight into the specific patterns of their infant's loss of contact? And what body interventions are useful in order to increase the parents' ability to respond when their baby is crying?

The current research status of EFA, as I present it here, has gone far beyond Reichian origins. Today, EFA combines the knowledge of modern body psychotherapy with findings of neurobiology (Porges 1998, 2005), psycho-traumatology (Levine 2010; Van der Kolk 2014) and attachment research (Bowlby 2010; Brisch 2000, 2013). The analysis of the mechanisms of parental contact ruptures, the emphasis on affective-cathartic expression processes on the part of the infant, as well as the inclusion of the therapist's psychosomatic resonance information, are still rooted in Reichian character analysis and bioenergetic research (Reich 1997). The emphasis on bodily self-observation, however, was inspired by awareness and trauma research (Ogden, Minton and Pain 2010; Siegel 2010; Weiss, Harrer and Dietz 2010). The increased focus on pre- and perinatal body language of the infant comes from the pioneers of prenatal psychology (Emerson 2012; Terry 2006, 2014). And the therapeutic relationship model prevalent in today's EFA is very similar to concepts used in humanistic psychology (Eberwein 2009; Eberwein and Thielen 2014).

Where can Emotional First Aid be applied?

This attachment-based body psychotherapy approach has three main areas of application. These three areas or 'pillars' (Figure 11.1) are:

- encouraging attachment

- crisis intervention

- parent–infant attachment psychotherapy.

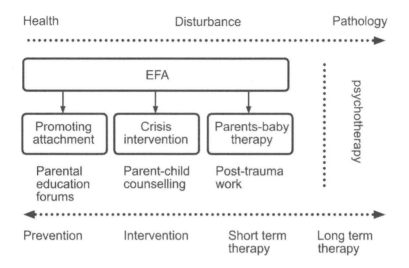

Figure 11.1 Three pillars of Emotional First Aid

Infants display an enormous capacity for change within psychotherapy, which is why in many cases only a small number of sessions are sufficient to remedy specific problems in the early development of the child. In the area of prevention, our work focuses mainly on coaching parents and children with a high level of resources and a strong ability to bond. Many parents seek answers to specific questions about how to handle their child's emotional outbursts, in particular their infant's crying. How long can one let a baby cry without him suffering damage? How should the child be held and positioned during crying? And what can parents do to prevent themselves from getting bound up by a current of raging emotions?

Often in EFA counseling, the goal is to show parents simple methods to regulate emotions, in order to enable them to stay in touch with their own body awareness during stressful moments in the relationship with their child. Prevention sessions consist of short psycho-educational units, during which the parents learn about the importance of bodily self-awareness and are taught simple breathing, imagination and perception techniques. Short videos demonstrate how to support a child during intense expression processes. In many cases, the main aim of these short interventions is for the parents to develop new ways of seeing and perceiving their child (Cierpka 2012).

The second pillar represents classical crisis intervention with parents, infants and young children who already display disturbances in emotional regulation when it comes to crying, sleeping and feeding. Here, interaction processes between parents and children have already suffered serious disruption. This is the main application area of EFA. Crisis counseling generally consists of three to six sessions, during which specific body intervention methods are applied in direct contact with the child. Through mindful self-observation or with specific changes in their breathing patterns, parents learn to better regulate their child's crying, and be with him through the crisis. The main aim of body psychotherapeutic crisis intervention is to strengthen the parents' ability to sense their child and resonate with him.

Many EFA counselors and therapists now work not just in specialized crisis intervention centers, but also within the context of clinical obstetrics and intensive birth assistance. Here, counseling sessions are held in the hospital at the mother's bedside, in the delivery room or in the neonatal care units.

The third pillar of EFA is directed towards parents whose ability to relate and regulate emotions has suffered as a consequence of pre-, peri- or postnatal trauma. In those cases, increasing the parents' sensitivity is not enough. Here, body-oriented parent–infant psychotherapy offers parents and children a space in which to recapitulate and integrate early relationship ruptures. Re-enactment of overwhelming experiences during pregnancy or birth, as well as separation traumas the family have not come to terms with, are of special significance in these situations. In later sections I will describe baby-centered work models in more detail (Evertz, Janus and Linder 2014; Schindler 2011).

Theoretical foundation of Emotional First Aid

Today's research in the field of EFA uses a attachment-based perspective for its therapeutic models. This is in accordance with other modern approaches within parent–infant counseling and psychotherapy which all focus on the reconstruction of a safe attachment relationship between parents and their children (Brisch 2000, 2010; Cierpka and Windaus 2007; Israel 2007; Papousek *et al.* 2004). The paths towards that goal, however, that is, the body-based concepts used in EFA, differ greatly from psychoanalytical or behavior therapeutic approaches of parent–infant therapy. Let us consider first the notion of attachment. What exactly do we mean by 'attachment' in the context of body psychotherapy with parents and babies? How can we integrate the classical term with the holistic, psychosomatic view as adopted in body psychotherapy?

As discussed in Chapter 2, the notion of attachment refers back to the research of the psychoanalyst and founder of modern attachment theory John Bowlby. He proved that the human need for closeness and intimacy is not the result of the child's oral-sexual needs, as assumed by psychoanalytical development theory. Bowlby considered the need for attachment as being a motivational system in its own right (Bowlby 1975). The need for closeness and intimacy is therefore just as important for the survival and thriving of a human being as the air we breathe and having enough food.

Attachment, according to Bowlby, is an invisible emotional connection through time and space between two or more people (Brisch 2010). Attachment represents a special form of relationship. Although attachment always means relationship, not every relationship allows for attachment. The most important characteristic is that the sustainable bond is a source of safety for the growing child. Successful attachment relationships are therefore a secure base that a person can refer to in moments of distress when they need support. It comes as no surprise that in times of great emotional need people do not refer to remote acquaintances such as their neighbors or members of their local sports club! In times of crisis, we look for emotional and physical support from those that we subjectively consider capable of providing us with a sense of safety.

For the infant, a safe attachment experience is a prerequisite for physical relaxation and letting go. Only the experience of the emotional availability of another allows the infant to withdraw his attention from the external world and refer back interoceptively to his own organism. At the same time, the repeated experience of attachment-based safety is an important condition that needs to be in place so that the infant can explore and feel comfortable in his environment.

From the perspective of the parents, a successful attachment relationship will contribute to their ability to decipher their infant's non-verbal body and behavior signals more accurately. Successful coherence or alignment with the child is felt as a sense of full bodily relaxation in the parents. Their breathing becomes deeper, their muscle tone lower and they have a calm heart beat.

From the perspective of body psychotherapy, physical relaxation and an ability to bond between parents and child are inextricably connected (Geuter 2015; Thielen 2009). Attachment and safety create openness and relaxation. Additionally, physical relaxation creates the fertile ground for successful attachment experiences. It is this connection that we make use of in parent–infant body psychotherapy.

The continuum and variability of parental attachment

The practice of body therapeutic crisis intervention allows us to closely observe the rapid changes in states of emotional regulation and attachment between parents and their child. The continuum stretches from very relaxed moments of connection between parents and infant to overwhelming feelings of threat, powerlessness and estrangement during times of rupture of the emotional bond. In this section we describe a phenomenological presentation of the individual stages of the parental attachment experience (Figure 11.2). What does a young mother feel when she is in close connection with her infant? And what happens physically and emotionally when the connection to the child is weakened or even ruptured during phases of increased stress?

Strong attachment	Weak attachment	Attachment breakdown
Safety	Threat	Threat to life
Relaxation	Mobilisation	Immobilisation
Attention alternates between contact with the self and contact with the world	Attention directed outward	Attention not focused
High self-connection	Weak self-connection	Loss of self-connection
Ventral vagus nerve	Sympathetic nervous system	Dorsal vagus nerve

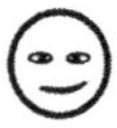

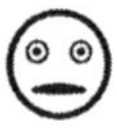

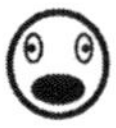

Figure 11.2 Continuum states of attachment

The state of reinforced attachment

When attachment and regulation capabilities are well developed, parents are able to move freely between times of contact with the child and moments of self-contact. The ability to align with, and tune into, the behavioral signals and needs of the child as well as being able to be aware of her own inner physical states are sufficiently developed. Physiologically, the mother is able to relax during calm contact with the child, for instance while feeding him. Her breathing flows easily and is deep and connecting. This ability to take deep breaths is a direct consequence of the relaxation of the diaphragm which, in turn, is a function of general opening and relaxation processes inside the body. The subjective experience in contact with the child is described in terms of safety, intimacy and well-being. Although the mother is intimately connected with the child, her attention rests with her own body. It is a simultaneous awareness of self and other.

This ability to self-observe allows the mother to check inwardly whether the interaction she offers her child is being experienced as 'right'. We are talking, in this context, about the parental ability to 'self-connect' (Harms 2008). Self-connection enables the parents to be co-regulators who are able to create and maintain an attentive connection with the stream of their own bodily and inner sensations. Attachment patterns as described in the context of attachment theory find their equivalent in similar patterns of safe, avoiding or ambivalent self-connection. Thus, building an internal and external 'relational thread' are two functionally identical processes within the parents' ability to provide stable and sufficiently safe attachment.

The state of weakened attachment

In the state of weakened attachment and ability to make coherent contact, those accompanying the child often have a sense of insecurity, lack of orientation and disconnection in the contact with the child. Often, these emotional states are exacerbated when attempts to soothe the infant during times of crying and restlessness fail. Important indicators of a growing spiral of stress and fear on the part of the parents are:

- increased muscle tension

- shallow breathing

- increased heart rate

- physical restlessness.

The focus of the parents' attention during those stressful phases shifts towards the crying child and the parents no longer manage to redirect their attention towards the inner sensations of their own body, even when the child is in a relaxed state.

Due to stress being generally dominant, the parents are less and less able to sufficiently grasp and guide the emotional expressions of their child. Quickly, a process of what is termed 'negative mutuality' arises: the child senses the stress-related loss of parental sensitivity and reacts with even more restlessness and crying (Papousek *et al.* 2004). This, in turn, intensifies the parents' insecurity and physical tension, and so on. Independently of the background and specific reasons for these regulatory and relational problems, the main aim of body psychotherapeutic intervention in EFA is to break this weakening vicious cycle as quickly as possible and return to a process of 'contagious health'.

In the above-described stress and alarm state, the parents still possess an ability, albeit limited, to maintain the connection inwardly and outwardly. Although all concerned experience a state of insecurity and tension, they are still able to perceive the 'real child' with all his needs. In this regulatory state within the therapy, they are also still capable of identifying and localizing inner physical and emotional clues such as 'each time little Johnny cries I've get a lump in my throat'.

The state of attachment rupture

The third regulatory stage in the parents' ability to bond occurs when, during contact with the infant, unprocessed trauma on the part of the parents is reactivated by the stress-triggering behavior of the child such as excessive crying fits, and chronic avoidance of eye contact. The intensity of stress and agitation in those phases is overwhelming and leads to a complete breakdown of the emotional connection with the child. Those involved find themselves trapped in a desperate state of powerlessness, unable to think, feel or act. While the baby lies crying in her mother's arms, the connection with the inner stream of bodily sensations disappears. This loss of self-connection on the part of the parent manifests in a sense of numbness, paralysis and the inability to focus.

During those dissociative episodes, the disconnection is twofold. On the one hand, those involved lose their capacity for introspection and self-awareness. On the other hand, their connection to, and sense of intimacy with, the 'real child' is lost. Fear of death as well as feelings of despair and hopelessness are nearly always present when parents experience these bottomless and totally unstable episodes of contact rupture with their child.

Attachment rupture, the loss of the ability to regulate emotions, as well as the collapse of bodily self-awareness, are inextricably interlinked during these phases of the attachment continuum. From the perspective of the child, the parental safety system collapses with the onset of dissociation.

Neuro-vegetative perspectives of Emotional First Aid

Now that we have a phenomenological description of the different regulatory states of parental attachment, I want to examine the physiological background of the parent–infant relationship and its disruption. Basic ideas and research can already be found in Wilhelm Reich's work, who saw the relational abilities of parents and children as deeply interwoven with the 'regulations' of the autonomic nervous system (ANS) (Reich 2010). Since these psycho-physiological findings, especially recent research regarding the ANS, are of fundamental importance for the concepts of EFA, I would like to briefly sketch them here.

The neuro-vegetative perspective of EFA is integrated with recent research by the American psychiatrist and psycho-physiologist Stephen Porges. His Polyvagal Theory offers an extensive set of explanations that help to underpin the previously described phases of the attachment continuum from a physiological point of view (Porges 1998, 2005, 2010). Furthermore, Porges' theory is useful for a more detailed representation of the effects of the specific body psychotherapeutic interventions within the parent–infant therapy. At the core of the Polyvagal Theory lies the hypothesis that the ANS contains three neuronal regulation circuits that create and maintain physical survival mechanisms.

According to the classical view of the ANS, the sympathetic nervous system and the parasympathetic nervous system consist of two branches.

Within the entirety of the human organism, they are responsible for a large number of inner organ functions that lie beyond the individual's conscious control. The parasympathetic system represents the 'rest branch' of the ANS. This system regulates regeneration and digestion and directs the attention inward so that energy resources can be replenished. The sympathetic nervous system, according to the traditional view of the ANS, mobilizes the body in order to counter threats. It activates the musculoskeletal system (fight or flight), means of expression (shouting, crying) as well as brain activity (efforts to find solutions). In the sympathetic stress and alarm state, we are highly alert and our attention is directed outward (Reich 2010).

The polyvagal point of view distinguishes itself from the classical one in that Porges considers the vagus nerve to be twofold (hence polyvagal). He differentiates between a younger branch of the vagal system, the ventral vagus, and an evolutionary older part of the vagus nerve, the dorsal vagus. The ventral vagus comes into action when we feel safe, warm and close to others. Under those conditions, it regulates our social orientation towards, and communication with, our most important attachment partners (Ogden *et al.* 2010). Turning our gaze towards others, spontaneous facial expressions, turning our head in the direction of the partner, and tuning of the hearing to the frequency range of the human voice are among the functions of the ventral vagus nerve.

This dominance of the ventral vagus system can be very clearly observed in the interaction between a mother and her baby. The mother seeks eye contact with the child, she smiles at him and repeatedly lifts her head, inviting the child to reciprocate her contact initiation. While talking to the child, her voice is of a slightly higher pitch (baby talk) and tuned to the child's auditive receptivity. Her facial expression is lively and open. Subjectively, feelings of safety, intimacy and well-being dominate the interaction.

From the point of view of evolutionary biology, the baby is programmed to begin the communicative exchange with his primary caregiver straight after birth. If the infant experiences those individuals as emotionally available on a regular basis, his ventral vagus system will be activated. The vagus dominance thus becomes the neuro-vegetative counterpart of the emotional experience of safety the child enjoys through the bond with those adults who care for him.

The polyvagal model describes a hierarchical order of specific neuronal regulatory circuits that serve to ensure survival. If the mother feels safe in her contact with the child, social exchange and mutual attachment are easy. If, however, her safe experience of attachment gets disrupted, the sympathetic stress and alarm system takes over. Typical parental stress indicators are hyperactivity (pacing up and down, inability to sit still, for example) along with increased perceptional tension and high thought activity (compulsive thinking, rumination). Only when strategies to avert the perceived threat fail will the evolutionary oldest regulatory circuit of the dorsal vagus with its 'shutting down mechanism' enter into action. In those existential emergency situations only inner organ systems are supported whilst energy is withdrawn from the periphery of the organism. This becomes very visible in shock paralysis when the legs go weak, the skin becomes pale and the individual is incapable of forming coherent thoughts.

Figure 11.3 shows the threefold autonomic nervous system based on Porges' model.

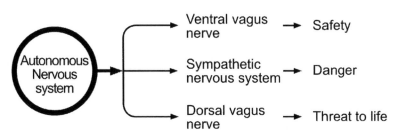

Figure 11.3 Threefold autonomic nervous system

Parental sensitivity and optimized windows of tolerance

From modern infant and attachment research we know that successful attachment relationships depend on the sensitive attunement between those caring for the child and the needs and behavioral reactions of the infant (Downing 2006; Siegel 2010). From the perspective of body psychotherapy, we can add that this sensitive parental competence requires an organism that has the ability to physically relax. Adults surrounding the child who are able to regularly enter a state of receptivity and openness are in a position to connect to the non-verbal signals of the child and adequately respond to them.

As we have described earlier, this mode in which the parents have the readiness to bond has its physiological foundation in the dominance of the ventral vagus function. The parents are able to react with calm and serenity to the various behavioral modes of the child. The successful attachment experience with its associated ventral vagus function inhibits the sympathetic stress and alarm reactions and dissociative trauma responses. In other words, the experience of attachment safety calms down the heart and respiration as well as the parents' raging thoughts. If the ventral vagus-based regulation maintains the experience of safety, 'negatively contagious' reactions, as are often observed between parents and their baby, do not occur. One could say that in this mode of openness the parents are like a lightning conductor for the stress reactions of their child. Severe phases of crying and restlessness during the night are tiring and exhausting, but the accompanying symptoms of hyper-excitation and threat, as can be seen in moments of crisis, no longer occur.

Whilst the parents remain in a state of openness and readiness to bond, the child can rely on their emotionally available presence during his quite draining phases of crying and restlessness. The parents act like a 'lighthouse' for their child. As long as the embodied self-connection of the parents is present, they represent an important support system that modulates the child's states of affective agitation. If, however, one or both parents are overwhelmed by the emotional impact, they will quickly leave this small window of tolerance that allows optimum attention to the infant. The child then loses his co-regulator. His crying remains unheard and the underlying needs and affective states no longer find the response they require. As a consequence, the quality of the crying becomes desperate and unending. If in those situations the parents are unable to build a bridge to the child, the stress and alarm mode of the infant will be replaced by one of resignation and emotional numbness. The child gives up and enters a state of paralysis. (See Figure 11.4 for activation levels of the autonomic nervous system.)

Within the neuro-vegetative view on attachment processes between parents and their newborns, all types of combinations are possible. A serene and emotionally available mother is there for her highly tense and alarmingly crying baby. Conversely, an inconsolable and angrily crying baby has a dissociated caregiver at his side; or perhaps a relaxed infant who is ready to bond meets with an adult caregiver who is emotionally insecure and unapproachable.

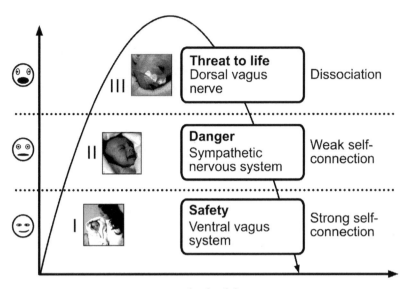

Figure 11.4 Activation levels of the autonomic nervous system

For the practice of EFA, these neuro-vegetative concepts represent an important diagnostic tool. During parent–infant body psychotherapy, based on the observation of body signals, the therapist is able to recognize whether those involved are leaving the narrow corridor of attachment availability. When, for instance, a young mother during a short interaction and observation phase suddenly starts fixating on her baby while her breathing becomes shallow and her posture becomes rigid, this indicates that the mother has lost her sense of safety in her connection with the child and is changing to a sympathetic stress mode. During therapy, this moment could be a first point of intervention where a deeper exploration of the mother's stress experience follows. As far as treatment goes, a number of questions arise from those findings:

- What can be done to prevent parents from permanently leaving their optimized attention and tolerance field in connection with their child?

- How can a body-psychotherapeutic procedure support parents so that they can either maintain or rebuild this narrow corridor of attachment availability during times of crisis?

The concept of self-connection in Emotional First Aid

As discussed earlier, the theoretical foundation of modern EFA is inextricably linked to the concept of self-connection. Historically, EFA's theoretical basis goes back to more recent research in the field of body psychotherapy (Davis 1999; Fogel 2013; Levine 2010) as well as models of awareness-based psychotherapy (Gendlin 1998; Weiss, Harrer and Dietz 2010). The main basis of the work, however, is clinical observations of applied body psychotherapy with parents and infants. In that context, it became obvious that initially used emotion-evoking techniques (e.g. deep breathing or expression exercises) and bioenergetic physical exercises were only partially useful when it came to helping them with the specific problems they were facing while trying to build a relationship with their baby (Harms 1999, 2008).

The analysis of postnatal crisis dynamics revealed that parents who lose the emotional connection to their newborn at the same time lose the connection to their own body sensations (interoception). So the loss of attachment comprises two sides of a single process: on the one hand, the loss of attunement with the infant; and on the other hand, the loss of contact with one's own bodily sensations. The most important core statement of EFA is that parental sensitivity requires a sufficiently stable self-connectedness. Secure self-connection means that the parent is able to revert back to his or her inner body and organ sensations. Conversely, loss of parental sensitivity always disconnects from the capacity for subjective experience and bodily perception (Fogel 2013).

Restoration of the parental ability to self-connect is therefore the most important core aspect of EFA methodology. This method enhances the known strategies used within depth-psychology and behavioral therapy when working with parents and children. The recovery of physical self-reference thus becomes the most important basis on which to modulate and change parental perception, thought and actions. By means of specific biofeedback systems, the parents are taught to become aware at a much earlier stage when they are on the verge of losing connection to their bodily self. One of the main ways of achieving this is the use of abdomen-focused breathing methods, which we refer to as abdominal breathing. By means of these methods, the parents learn to modify the stress-related weakening of their ability to regulate emotions in such a way that a rupture of alignment with and attunement to the child is prevented.

Self-connection therefore means that the parents possess the ability to maintain a double focus that enables them to stay in touch with themselves and with their child at the same time. The continual monitoring of the connection with their own breathing provides the parents with a diagnostic tool with which they can influence and regulate the quality of their attachment and their ability to make contact. Many parents put it this way: 'As long as I am in my belly, I am with my child' (Harms 2008).

Practically, establishing abdominal breathing achieves two important effects:

1. Continual self-awareness is maintained. By regularly checking whether she is 'still in her belly', the mother practices an important form of self-care. She cares about staying in touch with herself.

2. The use of abdominal breathing has an effect on the vagal branch of the autonomic nervous system that, in turn, initiates a number of regulatory circuits that will benefit the safe attachment process with the child. Among those effects are increased eye contact, relaxation of peripheral muscles, improved blood circulation in the skin, warmth being spread throughout the body, increased intuitive attunement with the child's affective needs, as well as an increased release of the attachment hormone oxytocin (Jansen and Streit 2015).

PRACTICE OF PARENT–INFANT BODY PSYCHOTHERAPY

Parental focus within Emotional First Aid crisis intervention

When parents bring their child for treatment, clinicians are often faced with a high degree of despair and helplessness on the part of the parents. The parents are under a lot of pressure due to attempted coping and solution strategies to deal with the child having failed over an extended period of time. Many parents report that they are no longer able to soothe their child with calming activities such as suckling (breastfeeding, bottle or a pacifier), lifting the baby, distraction, dancing or other movements, with these strategies being refused by the baby.

Depending on the severity of the parental distress, the therapist might feel high expectations at the beginning of the treatment with the assumption that solutions should be mainly directed towards the rapid relief of the child's manifest symptoms such as crying or sleeping problems. Parent–infant psychotherapists have to be very aware so as not to follow this immanent pressure on them to act.

Within EFA the specific interaction and attachment problems parents experience with their children are systematically explored and analyzed. I have extensively described this step-by-step procedure as the '7 step model' elsewhere (Harms 2000, 2008), but I want to summarize the most important aspects of this approach to crisis intervention below.

The opening phase of crisis interventions

After an initial phone call during which the parents explain their problem, they receive a questionnaire to be completed with the medical history of the child plus a cry-and-sleep journal. These details are brought along to the first treatment session. The questionnaire also gathers information about family members, the child's state of health, pregnancy and birth experiences as well as details regarding the parents' relationship with the child.

Especially when regulatory problems in the areas of crying and sleeping are present, a preliminary one-week journal which keeps note of time and duration of sleep and crying phases has proven to be very useful. Even prior to the therapy itself, this results in the parents being able to get a degree of objective perspective about the problem. Specifically, the extent of crying problems is often emotionally assessed and parents might describe their child's behavior in the following way: 'My baby has been crying for hours and hours at a time. This has been going on for weeks now. There is practically no let up.' The crying journal will correct this kind of perceptional distortion. The parents realize that their baby does not cry 'all the time' but at particular times, for instance always after breastfeeding or just before going to bed. Often, the parents are able to enter more into contact with the 'real child' during this one week's observation.

The first therapy session will serve to elicit important additional data about the different family members and the development of the child's symptoms to date. At the same time, the therapist is already able to discern important details in terms of body psychotherapy:

- How does the mother hold the child?

- What is her general emotional expression?

- What parental tension patterns can be observed?

- What is the emotional tone of their contact with the child? Is it warmhearted and sensitive or rather abrupt and aloof?

The way parents position their child gives many clues as to their level of sensitivity and the active attachment patterns: is the four-week-old baby held with his belly against the mother's body, his neck supported by his mother's hand, or does the mother, immediately at the beginning of the session, put the baby on the floor so that he is hardly able to make eye contact with his parents?

Clarifying the issue at hand and expectations of the therapy

Once the mother or parents have described their problem in a few sentences, we will try to assess together what their wishes and expectations are with regard to the course of the therapy session. Through empathic listening, the therapist will often be able to clearly discern what steps and goals are predominant. Four main therapeutic goals can be distinguished:

1. An improved attachment experience with the child

2. Improved general orientation when deciphering the child's behavioral language

3. Development of the parental ability to regulate emotions

4. Acquisition of concrete strategies for dealing with the child's difficult behavior such as crying phases in the evening.

Within the context of body psychotherapeutic crisis intervention, it is important to frame any expectations the parents have about the therapy process in small steps. This will enable an appropriate assessment of the therapy process at the end of the session. Are the results of the therapy session helpful in dealing with the concrete challenges the parents are faced with? Perhaps, at the end of the session, it might become clear that the session was enlightening because hitherto unreflected conflict processes within the family came into focus (e.g. transgression of boundaries on the part of an over-bearing mother-in-law). It is also possible that despite insights into the specific problems during the session, an improved ability to cope with the crying baby has not been achieved. It is then important that the parents realize this before the end of the therapy session and that it is taken into account when planning further sessions. When parents get the opportunity to voice any possible disappointment with the course of the therapy to date, early termination of the therapy can be avoided.

Observation of parental and infant behavior

During the first phase of treatment, the parents are invited to interact with their child in a natural and habitual way. Depending on the situation, it can be play, nappy change or feeding interactions that enable the therapist to observe the specific behavior the parents display towards their child.

The characteristic atmosphere that dominates the relationship between parents and child often unfolds within minutes. It is important to emphasize successful moments of interaction with the baby (for instance, exchanging a loving gaze, a sequence of physical touch) and bring them into awareness. Looking for positive aspects represents the most important guiding system during this initial treatment phase. We will often intensify the experience by inviting the parents to become aware of bodily sensations and localize them internally.

More severely affected babies often take only a few minutes before their behavior suddenly changes. Some of those babies suddenly change from an initial phase of relaxation and openness to restlessness. Others will enter a state of unexpected high-pitched crying. The nature of those behavioral changes are important markers in EFA intervention: first, they offer an opportunity to observe how the parents respond to the initial stress and expression process of the child; second, the subjective experience during these challenging moments with the child can be more clearly identified and named; and third, the parents can try out specific techniques to strengthen attachment and experiment with new behavioral strategies.

During this therapeutic exploration phase, the therapist is able to follow the parents' coping strategies. How exactly do they go about handling the child? For example, what are the individual steps in the parents' behavior before the crying escalates? Often repetitive and unconscious clusters of forms of behavior become visible. Those specific strategies are intimately related to the character and neurotic predispositions of the parents. It is important to allow this exploration to reach a point when the parents' hopelessness and loss of orientation typically begins (Downing 2006).

Body perception, internal exploration and somatic markers

When parents reach the point at which the strategies they use to deal with the problematic behavior of their child no longer work, agitation levels of all involved will quickly rise. Typically, behavioral sequences in contact with the child will speed up. Many parents will then cradle their child in a somewhat hectic way; the speech flow is more concentrated and faster. Everything in the parents' expression is accelerated. Furthermore, psycho-vegetative signals become visible, such as blushing, blotches on neck and breastbone, trembling and vibration of arms and legs, and breathing becoming faster and more shallow. So far, the parents might have seemed controlled and at a safe observational distance from the behavioral reactions of their child, but now their expression processes become stronger and more lively and the therapist is able to empathize. This tangible affective change in quality is a further turning point at which the therapeutic exploration is directed towards the subjective stress experience of the parents. The parents are being instructed to feel and name their conscious bodily sensations.

By focusing on the process of their bodily sensations, the parents are more easily able to adopt a non-judgmental attitude towards their inner experience. The goal of this approach is to link specific behavior patterns with patterns of bodily sensations. So, for instance, when the mother suddenly starts to cradle her child in a more agitated way, she might identify tightness in her abdomen. She feels how she holds her breath and how 'everything is being pulled into the upper body. It is as if I am no longer able to feel the lower half of my body and "forgot" it.'

This exploration of body sensation has a number of functions: first, it helps to recover the lost self-awareness of the parents; second, the conscious sensing of the body, similar to interoception, supports the individual's connectedness to reality. Bodily self-awareness creates a feeling of safety and orientation. The recovery of self-connection generates a self-strengthening cycle of relaxation and openness. At the same time, the baby benefits from the regained self-awareness. At the moment that the parents have reconnected with the information flow perceived from their own body and begin to feel themselves as a whole again, they become emotionally available and represent a safe ground for their child. The 'lighthouse' role of the caregivers is thus inextricably linked to adequate bodily self-perception and awareness (Fogel 2013).

Another important focus that plays a major role in future releasing strategies is the identification of different areas of the body – Damasio (2006) calls them 'somatic markers' – that are associated with weakening attachment experiences. In the example above, it is the tightness of the chest that represents the initial rupture in the contact with the child. These somatic markers serve as signaling systems that later on in the treatment can be used as early warning signs. The sensation of a tightening chest, for instance, tells the mother that the emotional connection with her child is in the process of being eroded. She can thus become aware of the fact that she is about to lose the emotional bond with herself and the child. This kind of bodily signal could serve as an identifiable signal in a state of agitation that specific stabilizing counter-measures are required.

Further body interventions that strengthen parental attachment availability

Modern body psychotherapy offers a whole array of specific tools to help parents regain a sense of safety and openness. Parallel to the previously described body awareness, EFA makes use of specific breathing techniques, physical touch and imagination exercises in order to support parental sensitivity and the ability to connect. I will now elaborate on a few of these interventions.

The use of physical touch to create safety

Physical touch in EFA is used to improve coherence and relational abilities. Before exploring areas of stress between parents and their child (whether those situations happen in real time or are being accessed through retrospective imagination), we ask the clients to indicate on what part of the body they would like to receive physical touch. This should be a place that they experience as stabilizing and strengthening. These so-called 'safety stops' are parts of the body that, when touched, trigger a maximum of attunement and connectedness. It is important that the individual experiences the touch in the most positive way possible. Particularly if the client has already entered a state of intense stress and alarm, they will experience the touch of a safety stop as extremely opening and safety-inducing. The touch initiates a process of generalized resonance and attunement that comprises affective, somatic, neuro-hormonal and behavioral aspects.

Seeing that the infant is normally present when the parents receive the touch, the induced affective attunement has an effect on the relationship between therapist and parents as well as that of each parent with their child (Harms 2008). Through the generation of a sense of safety, this specific touch enables the parents to reconnect with the inner sensations of their body. At the same time, the vagal regulation circuits that are responsible for the pro-social activities of the mother are being activated (Porges 2010). The mother is thus more in touch with herself whilst at the same time she begins to intuitively connect with the baby.

The use of supportive touch within the couple's relationship

One specific technique we often use in the context of attachment-based physical touch is to position the mother on the father's lap. The father is sitting on the floor whilst leaning against the wall. The mother sits on his lap and leans against his belly. The baby lies with his belly on the chest and belly of the mother.

This position allows mothers who are experiencing high stress levels during moments of crisis to physically feel a sense of closeness and support that is often missing in daily life. Most clients report that having their back supported helps them to let go of the need to control the situation and better tune into the needs and affective expressions of their child. In situations of extreme strain over a period of weeks and months (such as after long hospitalization due to a premature birth), this whole-body touch quickly opens up deeper emotional layers of the parents' self-awareness. Often the supportive touch of the partner opens the door to the expression of long-repressed emotions. Fathers also greatly benefit from this body-based experience of the relationship. Many report that, after long phases during which they were unable to act constructively, they regain the feeling of being useful and needed.

Physical touch in trauma-affected parents

The use of guided breathing processes is one of the most important interventions within EFA to specifically strengthen the parents' capacity for sensitivity and self-connection. The basis of this approach is the idea that initial states of stress and distress engage the activation of the sympathetic aspects of the autonomic nervous system. One of the main effects of dominant stress reactions is that the inhalation aspect of the breathing rhythm is emphasized. The diaphragm tightens and the breathing amplitude is reduced. A predominantly inhalation-based breathing pattern is often encountered when parents have been in stressful situations with their child for a long time (as in the care for excessively crying babies). EFA makes use of breathing patterns in various ways.

Breathing as diagnostic instrument

The observation of an individual's breathing pattern gives the therapist important clues as to their emotional state. If, during a massage session for instance, the mother holds her breath as soon as the child starts whining, this can possibly be a marker for an initial perceived threat on her part. The therapist then has the opportunity to draw the mother's attention to the stress-related change in breathing rhythm and then, through the exploration of the mother's body-awareness, the cause of the occurring tension can be clarified.

Breathing as modulator of the autonomic nervous system

By instructing the parents to adopt an abdominal breathing pattern, we encourage a counter-strategy. Abdomen-oriented breathing normally only occurs in situations of regeneration and safety. Consciously directed abdominal breathing assists the vagal branch of the autonomic nervous system, which, in turn, is responsible for the parents' intuitive behavior patterns (e.g. turning towards the child, modified tone of voice). The mother's attention to the physical perception of her abdominal breathing triggers a release of attachment-relevant hormones, an increase in skin temperature and relaxation of the peripheral muscles. Through resonance, the baby gets 'contaminated' by the mother's modified vegetative emotional state. The objective is thus to change vicious cycles into beneficial ones by means of altered breathing patterns (Papousek *et al.* 2004).

Breathing-assisted parental emotional safety

The recovery of self-connection quickly leads to alterations in the parents' prevailing mood. If they were unsure, hesitant and unable to make decisions before, access to embodied self-awareness now creates a foundation for the renewed experience of safety and general connectedness (towards the child as well as themselves).

Breathing as early warning system

In addition to the effects described above, the parents have the possibility to utilize the observation of their breathing as an important early warning system in the daily contact with their child. If the parents have a good grasp of the basic principle, this approach works astonishingly well. In many cases, the parents consider abdominal breathing a great help in all the everyday aspects of bringing up their child. On the one hand, they have a clear inner parameter to determine whether their availability towards the child is still present. On the other hand, they have an instrument at their disposal that allows them to counter any dysregulation or weakening of the sensitivity in their contact with the child.

Strengthening the readiness to bond by way of imagination

In EFA, we often encounter the problem that the difficulties the parents have with the child are not immediately observable within the therapy setting. This is particularly true for regulatory disturbances in the area of the child's sleep or, similarly, for situations of overwhelm during crying fits in the evening. Often, the baby will exhibit perfectly normal behavior during therapy sessions. In those cases, parent–infant psychotherapy will make use of imagination techniques in order to get closer to moments of strengthened attachment between parents and child. Here, the ability to visualize periods of successful attachment plays a particularly important role. The parents are invited to imagine a beautiful situation with their child and, while doing so, to observe their inner bodily reactions. For instance, imagining cuddling the child in the morning might lead to a feeling of widening of the chest together with a sense of happiness and contentment. Parents who have permanently lost the connection to their baby will find it difficult to remember the successful and positive moments with their child, although those are often still present. Positive imagination helps to attenuate negative self-judgment and enables a realistic new assessment of the concrete experience of the relationship with the child.

Similarly, imaginative approaches are used to create a state of 'safe' distance in order to observe problem situations more objectively. In this way, the focus continually switches between the external observation of behavior and the exploration of inner bodily and affective experiences. When the baby has fallen asleep on the mother's breast, she imagines the crying fits of her four-month-old son. She can see in her mind's eye how his imagined body expresses tension and distress. During imagination, the mother can grasp the concrete physical and affective signals of that situation by turning her attention to her body. She feels the tightness in her chest and the shallowness of her breathing. With the help of the therapist, she can link the bodily sensations of the 'now' with the stressful situations she experiences with her child in the evenings.

Another possibility is the connection of body-intervention techniques with imagination exercises. The mother is invited to direct her attention to the calm and expanding breathing movements in her body. Once she feels how warmth and relaxation spread through the body, the therapist invites her to take this abdominal breathing into the (imagined) stressful evening situation. Now the mother sees herself holding the crying baby in a serene attitude of connectedness. By linking imagination and bodily self-awareness, the client develops new practical perspectives in dealing with problem situations in daily life (Harms 2008).

A few remarks about body psychotherapy with fragile parents

We would like to point out that these specific body-therapeutic interventions are not always possible. If the parent is too depleted or the degree of their trauma too high, the use of touch and breathing can be counter-productive. In those cases, less emotionally focused approaches will be more adequate to support parents in the contact process with their child. Video-based interventions are one useful tool. The parents and the therapist watch successful interaction sequences that are subsequently discussed and analyzed in a positive way. The therapist has a twofold role when showing the video material (Downing and Ziegenhain 2001): on the one hand, he helps to describe and interpret the child's expressive behavior and its functionality;

on the other hand, he will emphasize the successful interaction and the resulting beautiful moments in the relationship between parents and child, thus drawing the parents' attention to those aspects (Cierpka 2012).

A further possibility, which we cannot elaborate on here, is to use successful interaction between the therapist and child as an example. Here, the therapist will lead the play or therapeutic touch with the infant while commenting on the child's expressive behavior, his specific perception of the child and the intention of his intervention in dialogue with the child. The objective is not so much a modification of the parents' mood and physiology but to cement the idea of other possibilities in terms of interaction.

The baby at the center of Emotional First Aid

Besides the body-oriented strengthening of the parents' relational sensitivity, direct body-psychotherapeutic work with babies themselves is a main characteristic that distinguishes EFA from other cognitive and behavioral parent–child therapies. The baby's behavioral reactions not only reflect the quality and the level of sensitivity in the parents' relationship with their child, they also place the child at the center of the therapeutic process. In the following, we describe the main models of baby-centered body psychotherapy as used within the concept of EFA.

Baby-centered bodywork

Babies suffering from regulatory disturbances display a high degree of bodily tension. Due to the acute stress, their ability to balance their emotions is limited on the vegetative level. Practically, many babies show paradoxical reactions: the parents' offering of touch and eye contact does not lead to relaxation and openness on the part of the child but instead triggers physical resistance, withdrawal and emotional outbursts. In this situation we use 'attachment through touch' (Deyringer 2008), a bonding-oriented development of a technique developed by Eva and Wilhelm Reich called 'butterfly touch technique'. This is an approach that invites the baby to gradually tolerate gentle skin and body touch. The main rule is to touch the infant only to the extent that he can remain in a state of openness. Duration, intensity and location of the touch have to be continually adapted to the child's ability to accept and tolerate it. For instance, even the gentlest touch of an infant's skull after extreme birth trauma such as vacuum extraction (ventouse) can trigger clear physical withdrawal and the avoidance of eye contact. The EFA therapist will reflect this stress reaction back to the baby and the parents with a phrase like: 'Ah, you do not like this. Now you are getting restless.' He will then move on to a different area of the body where touch is not experienced as a threat. During this body-centered interaction, the infant slowly regains trust and learns to enjoy full body touch again.

This approach is very effective in a number of ways. First, the babies experience a sense of safety and respect for their boundaries during the touch sequences. Astonishingly, even traumatized babies will quickly become mellow and return to a psycho-vegetative balance without the traumatic patterns having been activated (Meyer 2015; Wendelstadt 1999). One could say that this body-oriented method paves the way for successful moments of interaction between the baby and his parents, the positive experience being the healing agent. The main objective is a modification of the current vegetative reaction state. (See Figure 11.5.)

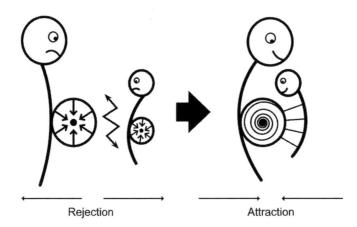

Figure 11.5 Self-connection and return to parental attachment activity

Second, through minimal tactile stimulation, the parents become aware of when and where they lose emotional connection with themselves and their child. Through the use of perception and breathing techniques, they also learn to sense insecurities as they arise and are able to modify them so that they can recover the 'relational thread' to their child. Third, during the guided massage sessions the parents can feel directly with their own hands how a very stressed baby will start to let go and relax physically. For parents who find emotional access to their child difficult, this is an especially effective way for them to notice the positive effect their touch has on their child.

Attachment-based support for the child's emotional outbursts

Another important aspect of the baby-centered work is paying attention to the infant's crying and outbursts that occur during therapy sessions. Our experience is that many babies have paradoxical reactions to the improved relaxation and contact shown by their caregivers. Often, short periods of openness are followed by a strong wave of emotional and physical expression. Suddenly, and often unexpectedly, the baby changes from a situation of clearly relating, to a stress state that includes intense crying. This is as a result of the improved self-connection and relational abilities of the parents creating the atmosphere in which hitherto repressed experiences of pain, powerlessness and existential distress can be expressed by the baby (Solter 2009).

Within EFA, paying attention to the infant's emotional expression process plays an important role. The aim of the 'assisted crying' process is to enable the parents to stay centered and strongly connected to their own body despite the strong emotional expression of their child. The previously described breathing, perception and touch techniques ensure that the parents are adequate 'containers' that can hold the baby's emotional expression. By maintaining their self-connection during a crying fit, the parents ensure that they do not get overwhelmed by unreleased 'ghosts' (Fraiberg 2011) and trauma from their own personal history.

Clinical observation has shown that babies are only able to come through their crying fits and enter a lasting state of relaxation if the parents maintain their self-awareness. The babies are usually being held against the parent's body during the crisis, but it is not the physical support that is decisive. It is the reconnection to self on the part of the adult caregiver that creates the relational foundation for the child to regain their lost emotional balance. During those attachment-based crying cycles, the babies go through a typical sequence of agitation and expression processes. I have described phases of the crying process in detail elsewhere (Harms 2008, 2013). To summarize, we can state that the baby-centered EFA crisis intervention aims at a transformation of the expressive quality of the child's crying. The baby feels, physically supported by his caregivers, the pain of previous ruptures in attachment and relationship. What is new, however, is that the babies now experience emotional connectedness during those regressions, which was not the case during the original pre-, peri- and postnatal ruptures.

It is often astonishing how quickly the expression and regulatory abilities of babies change after sessions of attachment-based expression assistance. Especially impressive is the fact that after the assisted crying crises, the children have far more ability to tolerate closeness to their caregivers and allow relaxation through physical touch.

Regressive approaches to pre-, peri- or postnatal trauma

As soon as the parents' co-regulatory abilities have been sufficiently developed, babies often start to 'tell the story' of their pregnancy and birth during therapy sessions. We then focus on the specific body language and expression processes of the child that give us clues as to the time and type of the pregnancy or birth trauma. In therapy sessions, infants spontaneously repeat the body postures that were linked to especially high stress points during the pregnancy or birth. Through body language they not only convey at what point it was 'too much' and what their distress was, but they also display what kind of support they would have needed in order to successfully complete the birth process by themselves (Hildebrandt 2015; Renggli 2013). During baby-centered process work, the therapist remains in constant dialogue with the child. He 'mirrors' the infant's body language and translates it into a language that allows the parents to view the origin of their child's problematic behavior (e.g. desperate non-stop crying) from a different and emotionally new perspective.

CASE STUDY

Daniel is four months old and was born by emergency Cesarean. During a therapy session he lies on his side during one of the observation sequences. He repeatedly starts a rotation movement. Although he has already learnt to roll from his back onto his belly, he suddenly stops and rolls back. His mother, who is watching, had been talking in detail about her pain and her 'stuckness' in the last phase of Daniel's birth. The child now rolls again onto his right side. He groans and a few moments later starts sobbing. He keeps turning his head from left to right as if he is trying to wrench himself away from something. His scalp is red and big drops of sweat appear on his forehead. I get the intuitive impulse to put my hand on the right-hand side of his skull. He now pushes his head into my hand and pushes against it. I start saying to Daniel: 'Yes, you are doing well. Show me what happened. I am with you.' I glance at the mother, who is following the process, and she, too, feels that her son is repeating and experiencing something important. I tell Daniel what I see: 'Your mother is also very close to you now and sees what is going on. Show us what happened and what your body wants to do.' Daniel's movements now become increasingly intense. I can see how he is struggling whilst pushing forward with his head. He is unable to get anywhere as if he was stuck. His crying is now desperate and high pitched. I keep encouraging the mother to connect with her child through the breath.

Suddenly, Daniel stops as if to take a creative break. With renewed momentum he successfully rolls onto his belly and starts to kick with his feet. I get the impulse to put my hands against the soles of his feet. Daniel is still sobbing but now he starts to push his legs vigorously, resulting in him moving across the mat in two or three movements. This is followed by a deep sigh on the out-breath. I now invite the mother to receive her son, who literally pushes himself into her hands. She picks him up and takes him into her arms. He is still breathing fast and is somewhat agitated. But it takes only a few moments for him to rest his head, relax his body and 'land' on his mother's belly. A few minutes of intimate silence pass. The room is filled with profound emotion and gratitude. The mother caresses Daniel gently and lovingly. 'Now I have the feeling that we are very close. I have never seen him like this,' she says at the end of the session.

Conclusion

This small case study is an example of birth regression. This baby-centered regression method has its place in EFA where the mothers and fathers have already gained the ability to self-connect securely. In this case, the infant relived an unfinished 'gestalt' of his birth process. However, the therapeutic benefit does not just consist in reliving and repeating a perinatal pattern. What matters most is that the baby experiences his parents as present and available co-regulators. Only newly felt relational safety creates the foundation for the infant to release and re-integrate specific developmental traumas.

I would like to conclude by emphasizing that within EFA, as opposed to other models of prenatal body psychotherapy, it is not the re-framing of overwhelming birth and pregnancy experiences that is the center of our focus. It is the development of an altered present-moment state that encourages embodied centeredness and emotional availability that this approach aims at (Stern 2010). The infant has to be able to feel the embodied experience of safety and being held. Developing embodied self-awareness on the part of the parents creates the necessary foundation on which implicit physical memories can be expressed and relived by the child. In my opinion, the benefit of this method does not so much lie in re-enactment but in the fact that, during the therapeutic regression of the child, the parents feel so safe within themselves that, even in the most difficult moments, they are able to 'stay with' their child.

References

Bowlby, J. (1975) *Bindung–Eine Analyse der Mutter-Kind-Beziehung*. München: Kindler.

Bowlby, J. (2010) *Frühe Bindung und kindliche Entwicklung*. München: Ernst Reinhardt.

Brisch, K.H. (2000) *Bindungsstörungen. Von der Bindungstheorie zur Therapie*. Stuttgart: Klett-Cotta.

Brisch, K.H. (2010) *SAFE. Sichere Ausbildung für Eltern*. Stuttgart: Klett-Cotta.

Brisch, K.H. (2013) *Schwangerschaft und Geburt. Bindungspsychotherapie – Bindungsbasierte Beratung und Therapie*. Stuttgart: Klett-Cotta.

Cierpka, M. (Hrsg.) (2012) *Frühe Kindheit (0–3 Jahre). Beratung und Psychotherapie für Eltern mit Säuglingen und Kleinkindern*. Heidelberg: Springer.

Cierpka, M. and Windaus, E. (Hrsg.) (2007) *Psychoanalytische Säugling-Kleinkind-Eltern-Psychotherapie. Konzepte – Leitlinien – Manuale*. Frankfurt a.M.: Brandes & Apsel.

Damasio, A. (2006) *Der Spinoza-Effekt. Wie Gefühle unser Leben bestimmen*. Berlin: List.

Davis, W.N. (1999) 'The Anorexic Adolescent.' In J.D. O'Brien, D.J. Pilowsky and O.W. Lewis (eds) *Psychotherapies with Children and Adolescents: Adapting the Psychodynamic Process*. New York: Jason Aronson.

Deyringer, M. (2008) *Bindung durch Berührung*. Berlin: Leutner.

Diederichs, P. and Jungclaussen, I. (2009) 'Zwölf Jahre Berliner SchreiBabyAmbulanzen – eine Positionierung körperpsychotherapeutischer Krisenintervention und früher Hilfen.' In M. Thielen (Hrsg.) *Körper – Gefühl – Denken*. Gießen: Psychosozial-Verlag.

Downing, G. (2006) 'Frühkindlicher Affektaustausch und dessen Beziehung zum Körper.' In G. Marlock and H. Weiss (Hrsg.) *Handbuch der Körperpsychotherapie*. Stuttgart: Schattauer.

Downing, G. and Ziegenhain, U. (2001) 'Besonderheiten der Beratung und Therapie bei jugendlichen Müttern und ihren Säuglingen – die Bedeutung von Bindungstheorie und videogestützter Intervention.' In H. Scheuerer-English, G.J. Suess and W.-K. Pfeiffer (Hrsg.) *Anwendung der Bindungstheorie in Beratung und Therapie*. Gießen: Psychosozial-Verlag.

Eberwein, W. (2009) *Humanistische Psychotherapie. Quellen, Theorien und Techniken*. Stuttgart: Thieme.

Eberwein, W. and Thielen, M. (Hrsg.) (2014) *Humanistische Psychotherapie. Methoden, Theorien, Wirksamkeit*. Gießen: Psychosozial-Verlag.

Emerson, W. (2012) *Behandlung von Geburtstraumata bei Säuglingen und Kindern*. Heidelberg: Mattes.

Evertz, K., Janus, L., and Linder, R. (2014) *Lehrbuch der Pränatalen Psychologie*. Heidelberg: Mattes.

Fogel, A. (2013) *Selbstwahrnehmung und Embodiment in der Körperpsychotherapie. Vom Körpergefühl zur Kognition*. Stuttgart: Schattauer.

Fraiberg, S. (Hrsg.) (2011) *Seelische Gesundheit in den ersten Lebensjahren*. Gießen: Psychosozial-Verlag.

Gendlin, E. (1998) *Focussing – orientierte Psychotherapie. Ein Handbuch der erlebnisbezogenen Methode*. München: Pfeiffer.

Geuter, U. (2015) *Körperpsychotherapie. Grundriss einer Theorie für die klinische Praxis*. Heidelberg: Springer.

Harms, T. (1999) 'Instroke und frühe Säuglingsentwicklung. Theorie und Praxis der bioenergetischen Säuglingsforschungen Wilhelm Reichs.' In H. Lassek (Hrsg.) *Wissenschaft vom Lebendigen*. Berlin: Leutner.

Harms, T. (Hrsg.) (2000) *Auf die Welt gekommen. Die neuen Babytherapien*. Berlin: Leutner.

Harms, T. (2008) *Emotionelle Erste Hilfe. Bindungsförderung, Krisenintervention, Eltern-Baby-Therapie*. Berlin: Leutner.

Harms, T. (2013) 'Eltern-Baby-Körperpsychotherapie im Spannungsfeld von Trauma und Bindung.' In M. Thielen (Hrsg.) *Körper – Gruppe – Gesellschaft. Neue Entwicklung in der Körperpsychotherapie*. Gießen: Psychosozial-Verlag.

Hildebrandt, S. (Hrsg.) (2015) *Schwangerschaft und Geburt prägen das Leben*. Heidelberg: Mattes.

Israel, A. (Hrsg.) (2007) *Der Säugling und seine Eltern. Die psychoanalytische Behandlung frühester Entwicklungsstörungen*. Frankfurt a.M.: Brandes & Apsel.

Jansen, F., and Streit, U. (Hrsg.) (2015) *Fähig zum Körperkontakt*. Heidelberg: Springer.

Levine, P. (2010) *Sprache ohne Worte. Wie unser Körper Trauma verarbeitet und uns in die Balance zurückführt*. München: Kösel.

Meyer, A. (2015) *Sanfte Schmetterlings-Babymassage*. Frankfurt a.M.: Meyer-Info3.

Ogden, P., Minton, K., and Pain, C. (2010) *Trauma und Körper. Ein sensumotorischer orientierter psychotherapeutischer Ansatz*. Paderborn: Junfermann.

Overly, R.C. (2005) *Gentle Bioenergetics. Theory and Tools for Everyone*. Greensboro, NC: Lifestyle Press.

Papousek, M., Schieche, M., and Wurmser, H. (2004) *Regulationsstörungen in der frühen Kindheit*. Bern: Huber.

Porges, S. (1998) 'Love: An emergent property of the mammalian autonomic nervous system.' *Psychoneuroendocrinology 23*, 8, 837–861.

Porges, S. (2005) 'Neurozeption – die drei Regelkreise des Autonomen Nervensystems.' In *Trauma-Newsletter*. Zürich: Zentrum für Innere Ökologie.

Porges, S. (2010) *Die Polyvagal-Theorie. Emotion. Bindung. Kommunikation und ihre Entstehung*. Paderborn: Junfermann.

Reich, E. and Zornànszky, E. (1993) *Lebensenergie durch Sanfte Bioenergetik*. München: Kösel.

Reich, W. (1987) *Children of the Future. On the Prevention of Sexual Pathology*. New York: Farrar, Strauss & Giroux.

Reich, W. (1997) *Charakteranalyse*. Köln: Kiepenheuer & Witsch.

Reich, W. (2010) *Die Entdeckung des Orgons I. Die Funktion des Orgasmus*. Köln: Kiepenheuer & Witsch.

Renggli, F. (2013) *Das goldene Tor zum Leben: Wie unser Trauma aus Geburt und Schwangerschaft ausheilen kann*. München: Arkana.

Schindler, P. (Hrsg.) (2011) *Am Anfang des Lebens. Neue körperpsychotherapeutische Erkenntnisse über unsere frühesten Prägungen durch Schwangerschaft und Geburt*. Basel: Schwalber-Verlag.

Siegel, D.J. (2010) *Die Alchemie der Gefühle*. New York: Kailash.

Solter, A. (2009) *Warum Babys weinen. Die Gefühle von Kleinkindern*. München: Kösel.

Stern, D. (2010) *Der Gegenwartsmoment: Veränderungsprozesse in Psychoanalyse, Psychotherapie und Alltag*. Frankfurt a.M.: Brandes & Apsel.

Terry, K. (2006) 'Therapeutische Arbeit mit »Schreibabys«.' In G. Marlock and H. Weiss (Hrsg.) *Handbuch der Körperpsychotherapie*. Stuttgart: Schattauer.

Terry, K. (2014) *Vom Schreien und Schmusen, Vom Weinen zur Wonne: Babys verstehen und heilen*. Wien: Axel Jentzsch Verlag.

Thielen, M. (Hrsg.) (2009) *Körper – Gefühl – Denken. Körperpsychotherapie und Selbstregulation*. Gießen: Psychosozial-Verlag.

Van der Kolk, B. (2014) *Verkörperter Schrecken. Traumaspuren in Gehirn, Geist und Körper und wie man sie heilen kann*. Lichtenau: G.P. Probst Verlag.

Weiss, H., Harrer, M.E., and Dietz, T. (2010) *Das Achtsamkeitsbuch. Grundlagen, Anwendungen, Übungen*. Stuttgart: Klett-Cotta.

Wendelstadt, S. (1999) 'Heilung durch Berührung. Eva Reichs Baby-Schmetterlingsmassage zur Erhaltung der Gesundheit und Vorbeugung von Biopathien.' In *Emotion, Band 14*. Berlin: VKD-Publikationen.

CHAPTER 12

THERAPIES FOR BABIES AND CHILDREN

John Wilks

Introduction

This chapter describes a selection of treatment options available for babies and children. It is by no means exhaustive. Some therapies have been around for longer than others and some are more aligned to current understandings about neurology, development, trauma and pre- and perinatal psychology than others.

Touch is an important part of any therapeutic approach for babies, and most therapies can be adapted to use with babies. Acupuncturists will usually use touch instead of needles, and there are various other therapies such as Bowen, infant massage, shiatsu, reflexology, osteopathy, aromatherapy, homeopathy, herbal medicine and naturopathic approaches which can all be useful. For the toddler, working therapeutically with primitive reflexes can also be invaluable as they go through important developmental milestones.

We start with Cranial Osteopathy as it has probably the longest pedigree of all therapies applied to babies and children apart from Traditional Chinese Medicine. Biodynamic Craniosacral Therapy is given a separate section here as it is used by both osteopaths and other therapists and has a particular orientation when working with babies. Other therapies are given briefer outlines as they tend to be used to address specific behavioural, postural or developmental issues. Having read this far, the potential limitations of using a purely biomechanical approach to working with babies and children will hopefully have become apparent. The range of skills outlined in this book can be used by any therapist and will greatly enhance any techniques they use.

PART 1: MANUAL THERAPIES

Cranial Osteopathy[1]

Cranial Osteopathy is a very gentle but immensely powerful form of treatment, ideally suited to the treatment of babies and children. On the one hand, it is possible to witness the immediate unravelling of retained moulding patterns following a prolonged or traumatic delivery. On the other, treatment given to an infant that was premature, or who had a very rapid arrival into this world, may have no visible indicators but can help that individual become 'at one' with themselves, can give them better centring and allow them to have ownership of the space they occupy; this may help them to cope better with any temporary separation from the maternal space.

Feeding difficulties are an example of an issue which is best resolved with cooperation across many disciplines. Lactation consultants give invaluable advice regarding positioning and can also resolve issues around tongue-tie. Osteopaths can ensure good movement of the head and neck: if feeding is easier on one side than the other, it might be that a difficult rotation through the birth canal has locked one of the condyles where the skull sits upon the top of the neck. This prevents the baby from looking comfortably to one side or the other. Another factor considered by an osteopath would be trauma to the jaw, especially after a forceps delivery or face presentation. The lower jaw (mandible) should swing freely from the temporomandibular joint permitting easy movement both up/down and forward/backward. Without this jutting movement of protraction, baby will not be able to milk the nipple efficiently, even if the tongue is fully functioning. Protraction is essential to form a good lip seal and to enable a drop in intra-oral pressure so that the milk can be extracted: just chomping up and down is not good enough and can be very painful for mother. The position of the palate is also vital; ventouse extraction places strong forces upon the vault and the delicate membranes of the skull and can sometimes be felt as a raised, narrow palate. Balancing the tension can allow the palate to broaden and lower so that the tongue can more easily milk the nipple against the roof of the mouth.

The roof of the mouth is also the floor of the nose: perhaps baby is having difficulty in sustaining the act of feeding because he can't breathe freely.

---

1   This section on Cranial Osteopathy has been written by Anita Hegerty.

The act of breastfeeding is hard work. It needs clear nasal passages and coordinated, rhythmic suckling and swallowing. An osteopath can open up the face, easing tension between the delicate bones and thus allowing easier breathing. This has ongoing benefits: prolonged mouth breathing has been shown to have profound long-term effects on postural development of the head and neck, positioning of the jaw (giving a retracted 'weak' chin) and dental alignment.

Another factor to consider when there are feeding issues is the function of the tongue: tongue-tie may be snipped, but if the back of the tongue is held in tension then baby will still be unable to extend the tip of the tongue forwards. Osteopathic treatment to the delicate structures of the throat and under the chin can ensure release of this area; especially relevant if there have been issues of the cord around the neck or difficulties during early breathing.

'Cranial' Osteopathy is not applied just to the head. It is a treatment technique which works on the primal rhythm; this starts at the cranium but it extends to all parts of the body. A case study involving a little girl with mild developmental delay illustrates this well: at 20 months old she was still not walking; the upper extremities met all the expected milestones – hands to the midline, hands to mouth, reaching, grasping and manipulating objects, and so on. Development of the lower extremities, however, had not followed the same timeline: there had been a delay in the ability to sit unsupported; quadruped crawling did not occur but was replaced by commando crawl whenever she wished to get anywhere. Pushing up to standing, creeping and assisted walking were all hard to achieve and each seen as a major event. Her mother lamented that I missed each progressive step because it seemed to occur just after our scheduled appointment. I was thrilled, however, that this was the case: each came about after a treatment when I had been able to look at the function of the sacrum, the lumbar plexus of nerves, the lumbar enlargement of the spinal column and the balance of the pelvis; contact on the lower back and sacrum gave a fulcrum around which health and healing could be expressed. The supportive contact enabled the pelvis to reorganize, remove the restriction and enable the neurological system to express the next phase.

Another fascinating area of integration is speech therapy. Vocalization requires the lips, tongue and jaw to work independently of one another. The factors essential for good breastfeeding also work to shape the sounds. Speech also requires a mature breathing pattern which allows a steady, slow and sustained release of air and controlled intra-oral pressure. This three-dimensional respiratory action requires good rib activity, appropriate diaphragmatic tone, strong back and abdominal muscles plus gentle soft-tissue recoil. No wonder we don't learn to speak until after we can hold ourselves upright! Osteopathic assessment of thoracic function supports good respiratory function through release and support of the mechanics.

Osteopathy may also unlock early shock held in the tissue memory of the diaphragm/umbilicus or in the peripheral skeleton. Emotional and physical trauma can be locked into tissues for many years. If it is unresolved it may surface years later when the tissues are placed under increased demand. This might be at puberty when growth and skeletal shape change alter tensions within the structure. Or it might be later in life when a second trauma unlocks the expression of an injury sustained long ago. Or it might even become expressed when a child starts to be fitted with orthodontic braces; locking the structure at one site causes the retained patterns to be expressed at another. Alternatively, the holding pattern may remain fixed and lead to strained patterns of posture, breathing and digestion, causing a lifetime of compromised function, depleted energy and susceptibility to illness. W.G. Sutherland, the founder of Cranial Osteopathy, expressed this phenomenon when he coined the phrase 'as the twig is bent, so the tree will grow'.

Biodynamic Craniosacral Therapy

Craniosacral Therapy developed from the work of W.G. Sutherland, himself a student of A.T. Still, the founder of osteopathy. It has been taught to non-osteopaths for nearly half a century, and craniosacral therapists use a variety of approaches. These may incorporate an understanding of trauma, embryological development and pre- and perinatal psychology. The term 'biodynamic' refers to an approach that was developed by Franklyn Sills, where the body is encouraged to respond to expressions of its own ordering blueprint. Nothing is imposed from the outside; rather, inner health and vitality (sometimes referred to as 'potency') is encouraged to express itself, affecting not only the bones and tissues but also the nervous system, allowing restrictions, held trauma and emotional issues to resolve at their own pace.

Craniosacral therapists work with various 'tide-like' movements expressed through the tissues and fluids of the body. These tides provide a reference point to health and are sometimes referred to as the cranial rhythmic impulse (8–14 cycles per minute), the mid-tide or fluid tide (2.5 cycles per minute) and the long tide (one cycle every 100 seconds). Because Craniosacral Therapy is so gentle, it is particularly suited to use with babies.

Craniosacral Therapy and breastfeeding[2]

There is much research about the general health benefits of breastfeeding, including protecting the baby from gastroenteritis, allergies, eczema, asthma, urinary tract infections, bronchiolitis, diabetes and sudden infant death syndrome, to name but a few. It also offers the baby pain relief as it is packed with beta endorphins, particularly if the mother has experienced pain in labour. The benefits to the mother include protection against breast cancer, ovarian cancer and osteoporosis. Breastfeeding works in harmony with the hormones associated with bonding to support a healthy attachment for mother and baby.

For a baby to be able to feed well at the breast he/she should be able to come to the breast in a position that enables effective milk transfer. Ideally the baby should be able to reach up to the nipple, open their mouth widely and take a good amount of the nipple and surrounding areola. The baby should then be able to form suction on the nipple and pull it back to the junction of the hard and soft palate; this will enable the baby to work the milk ducts within the breast and remove the milk using a rolling action of the tongue. The baby should be able to organize a suck–swallow–breathe pattern which leads to relaxed, comfortable feeding for both mum and baby.

After birth, babies generally spend the first couple of hours awake. This is a very special time as the baby sees mum and dad for the first time and adjusts to life outside the womb. Once their adrenaline levels begin to drop, the baby begins to explore her immediate environment by touching and licking. This encourages early feeding behaviours and the baby will start to seek the breast. This first feed is unique and instinctive; the baby will go on and off the breast frequently during this feed to build muscle memory and develop brain pathways around how to feed at the breast.

Here the first challenge to breastfeeding may begin. Many babies will be born under the influence of pain relief given to their mums during labour.

---

2   This section on Craniosacral Therapy and breastfeeding has been written by Kate Rosati.

Both pethidine and epidurals can cross over to the baby and make her sleepy; this sleepiness may last for 24 hours or more after birth, meaning that she misses the first instinctive feed. Babies who have had a difficult birth (including elective Caesarians) may have high levels of adrenaline for longer and be unable to seek the breast, or quickly fall asleep as a way of coping with their experience. These babies may well have experienced unequal pressure on their skulls during birth which can lead to pain, bruising and oedema. It is common to see these babies refuse to feed or position themselves to protect the areas that hurt.

Common breastfeeding problems

Generally babies come for craniosacral sessions from two weeks of age, but by this time compensatory patterns of feeding may well be present and causing problems. Some examples of this are listed below:

- Baby prefers to feed on one breast rather than the other or in one position.

- The baby does not draw the nipple back to the soft palate, which causes soft tissue trauma to the nipple.

- Fussing at the breast.

- Baby does not open the mouth widely at the breast; this can lead to fussing at the breast and can affect the amount of milk the baby is able to remove and the amount of fat transferred with the milk.

- The baby may be unable to open its mouth widely, therefore limiting the amount of breast tissue taken into the mouth when feeding. This can lead to reduced milk transfer.

- Being reluctant to go to the breast in the first place.

- Being unable to form a suction once attached to the breast.

- Struggling to swallow the milk once the let down happens.

- Unable to transfer milk from a full breast.

- The baby never seems satisfied and wants to suck a lot.

If feeding problems continue, the mum's milk supply may reduce, causing weight loss and failure to thrive.

It is easy to put the above problems down to a new mum and baby learning experience; however, over time I have become more curious about this, especially when feedback after a Craniosacral Therapy session often includes improvements in feeding. For a baby to feed effectively at the breast the baby needs to be willing and able to feed, and specifically to have no respiratory issues, as breathing over-rules sucking.

The neonatal skull

To understand why birth may affect the way the baby feeds at the breast we first need to look at the structure of a baby's skull and what happens to it as it passes through the pelvis during birth. During labour the environment of the uterus changes; the force of the contractions travel down the baby's spine along the longitudinal axis with the intention of pushing the baby forward, but the cervix and pelvic anatomy act as a barrier and create resistance to the head. The forces of normal labour are significant: 60–85 Hg/167–236 pounds per square foot. The combination of these two forces coming together often causes pressure through the neck and cranial base, giving rise to an area of compression. These forces have the potential to compress sections of the bones, leading to irritation or activation of the cranial nerves that exit through the cranial base.

The cranial nerves

There are a number of nerves that exit the jugular foramen next to the jugular vein. If distortion has occurred in this area from compression during birth, the operation of these nerves can be affected. It is also possible that venous return within the jugular vein is slowed, resulting in oedema which could also affect these nerves.

The *vagus* nerve has an influence on the larynx, heart, lungs, trachea, liver, gastrointestinal tract and digestive function. It coordinates sucking with breathing, vital for effective milk transfer and comfortable feeding. Disruption with the efficient functioning of this nerve has been linked to colic and reflux.

The *accessory* nerve innervates the sternocleidomastoid and trapezius muscles. These muscles stabilize the baby's head, allow the movement of flexion and rotation, and maintain an open airway. Activation or irritation of this nerve may lead to the baby having reduced movement on turning their head, leading to feeding only being possible in one position. A compromised airway will affect the suck–swallow–breathe coordination.

The *glossopharangeal* nerve also exits through the jugular foramen and acts on the posterior one-third of the tongue and the stylopharyngeus muscle, which when stimulated elevates the pharynx during swallowing. Irritation of this nerve may lead to reflexive guarding of the airway by the tongue pressing upwards onto the palate. Tongue thrusting prevents deep attachment at the breast, which can lead to soft tissue damage of the nipples. This nerve is also involved in the initiation of the gag reflex; if the baby has a hyper-responsive gag reflex it may be difficult for the baby to draw the nipple back to the junction of the hard soft palate, which is the position required for comfortable feeding.

The *hypoglossal* nerve exits through the hypoglossal canal situated in the condylar part of the occiput (see Figure 10.1). This nerve acts on the tongue muscles, allowing the tongue to make the stripping action needed to draw milk from the breast. Irritation of this nerve may lead to a compromised tongue action affecting the movement forwards or backwards or cause the tongue to deviate off to one side of the mouth.

The *trigeminal* nerve innervates muscles that control the mouth actions of opening, closing and sucking. For optimal attachment to the breast the baby's mouth needs to open around 160 degrees.

The motor branches of the *facial* nerve innervate the facial muscles, lips, cheek and jaw, which initiate the rooting, latching and sucking responses. If this nerve is compromised, the baby may use his lip muscles rather than tongue and intra-oral muscles to suck, which will affect the suck–swallow–breathe coordination and the comfort of a feed experienced by mum.

How the baby tries to correct compression within the cranial base

Babies have strategies to try and correct compression within the cranium. The first breath increases the intracranial pressure, thus expanding the cranium and repositioning the bones of the skull. However, some bones may be too stuck, or the first breath not deep enough for this to make a significant difference, so the baby may have to resort to plan B. By crying, sucking and yawning, intracranial pressure is again increased in a bid to give the cranial bones more movement.

Anatomically, by sucking, the baby stimulates a bone called the vomer, which runs just above the bones of the palate. This bone effectively acts as a cog in relation to other cranial bones, helping to free them up through a rhythmical rocking motion generated by the baby's sucking action, and gives space to the structures which house the cranial nerves.

How craniosacral therapy can help

Parents often bring their babies for treatment because they are struggling and looking for help. Craniosacral therapists have a wonderful opportunity to educate and support parents, to bring awareness and empathy to these symptoms and to recognize them for what they are rather than seeing the baby as naughty, manipulative or controlling.

Sitting and observing a baby, paying attention to the baby's breath and movements, will give the therapist an idea of the holding patterns and how to work with them. A digital examination of the mouth gives information about how the baby uses her tongue and how the bones of the palate are aligned. Paying attention to the gag reflex and noticing how much contact the baby needs on the palate to stimulate the suck reflex also gives information about how the baby behaves whilst feeding.

Listening to a baby whilst they are feeding gives an insight into how they are able to coordinate themselves, paying attention to the quality and tension of the breath, the rhythm and sound of the swallow, and noticing any pauses. The pauses are important to allow the baby to catch her breath and rest the muscles before going for another burst.

Generally babies are very quick to respond to treatments; within only a couple of sessions, the feedback shows how much the family have relaxed. When breastfeeding is going well, everyone is happy!

Bowen Technique

The Bowen Technique is a relatively new therapy, but it is rapidly gaining popularity in treating babies and children with some remarkable results. Bowen is very 'light touch' and can be extremely helpful for babies who are unsettled, fractious or colicky. Some simple steps that parents can use at home are outlined in Carolyn Goh's online book at www.babybowen.com. Bowen is also offered at a number of low-cost clinics throughout the UK. Details can be found in the Resources section later in this book.

Bowen mainly works by a therapist applying light pressure and gentle 'rolling' type moves to the connective tissue and fascia. This can help free up areas of the body such as a tight diaphragm or a neck restriction but also has a profound relaxing effect on the nervous system. It can also be used to help with sleeping, feeding, digestive and developmental issues such as crawling.

There are specific Bowen moves that work on babies' diaphragm and psoas muscles which can give almost instantaneous release from symptoms such as colic and reflux. Because the psoas has attachments at the back of the diaphragm, any tightness here will tend to affect breathing as well as the structures that pass through the diaphragm (e.g. the oesophagus and lower branches of the vagus). Bowen practitioners also work on the TMJ, which has a profound effect on the hard palate and alignment of the jaw; something that can cause feeding, speech and later dental problems unless it is addressed. My book *Using the Bowen Technique* describes remarkable projects using Bowen for digestive and bowel problems, asthma and problems with excessive mucus.

Infant and baby massage

Baby massage can be a wonderful and relaxing way to encourage bonding between mother and baby. Anita Hegerty writes:

> Although one generally thinks of massage as a means to relaxation, occasionally it needs to be stimulating: premature babies, or babies with special needs, can have floppy muscle tone. Massage applied correctly can invigorate the nerve endings and lead to better muscle tone throughout. Physically, massage increases the circulation and improves the lymphatic drainage. Increased circulation and lymphatic function can help the immune

system to develop. It can also give improvement in breathing and digestive function, helping to ease mucus drainage, colic, flatulence and constipation.

There has been some suggestion that regular, non-threatening and loving, physical touch can reduce the hypersensitivity induced by noxious events around the birth process. If baby has had intensive medical investigations or interventions in the early hours/days of life, then slow, gentle massage conducted in a quiet environment can reverse the association of touch and pain; it can calm the nervous system, reduce the 'startle' response and improve sleep patterns.

PART 2: PSYCHOTHERAPEUTIC AND INTEGRATIVE APPROACHES

Integrative Baby Therapy

Integrative Baby Therapy draws from a number of sources discussed in this book including pre- and perinatal psychology, body psychotherapy and Craniosacral Therapy. It is also informed by recent research in areas such as self-regulation, neurobiology, epigenetics, biodynamic embryology, field theory, attachment theory, traumatology, consciousness research and cross-cultural studies.

Filial Therapy and Play Therapy

Filial Therapy was developed in the 1960s and is a very adaptable type of Play Therapy suitable for children between the ages of 3 and 11. Filial Therapy's core principle is to encourage parents to learn the necessary skills to become therapeutic agents in their children's lives, providing them with training in basic Play Therapy techniques so they can use these techniques at home. Trained professionals educate parents usually over a two-week period in the method and then provide supervision and guidance as families begin to integrate it into their lives.

Equine Assisted Therapy

There are two main types of Equine Assisted Therapy that have been used for over 40 years: one related to education and learning and the other using more of a psychotherapeutic and physical therapy approach. Equine therapy can be very helpful for children suffering from ADHD, attachment issues and anxiety. It can also help children improve their cognitive, physical, emotional, social and behavioural skills and is usually a combination of many horse-related activities. On a physical level, a horse's movements stimulate the rider's muscles which benefits patients suffering from physical disabilities, and influences the systems responsible for speech production. It impacts the muscles involved with breathing and can assist respiratory function. There is a lot of research available on Equine Assisted Therapy related to mental health at http://equineassistedinterventions.org.

Dyadic Developmental Psychotherapy (DDP)

DDP was developed by the psychologist Dan Hughes as a method for working with adopted or fostered children and their families. The DDP approach integrates attachment theory, developmental trauma, the neurobiology of trauma, caregiving and child development. Adoption presents specific challenges as adopted or fostered children often find it hard to trust adults. They may have problems with creating secure attachments to their adopted parents and try to stop their new parents from becoming emotionally close to them.

Central within the DDP approach is Playfulness, Acceptance, Curiosity and Empathy (PACE), all of which aim to deepen emotional connections to others. The therapy helps the children learn to trust. It is family-based and involves the child with his or her caregivers.

Theraplay

Theraplay is a fun way of developing attachment, assisting development and encouraging a sense of safety. In a Theraplay session the therapist guides the parent and child through playful, fun games, and developmentally challenging activities. The act of engaging in this way helps the parent regulate the child's behaviour and helps him feel secure, cared for, and connected. Theraplay encourages four of the essential qualities found in parent–child relationships: structure, engagement, nurture and challenge. The purpose of Theraplay sessions is to increase the emotional connection between a child and his parent, engendering a changed view of the self as worthy and lovable and of relationships as positive and rewarding.

Family Constellations Therapy

Family Constellations Therapy was pioneered by the controversial psychotherapist and philosopher Bert Hellinger in the 1970s, and is an approach aimed at helping to reveal and heal hidden dynamics in a family or relationship. A family constellations session usually takes place within a workshop setting but can also work within a therapeutic one-to-one session. Other therapists have since developed Hellinger's work further into the fields of Systemic and Organizational cultures to solve relationship problems within and between individuals and organizations.

With particular respect to the theme of this book, constellations have been further refined and developed through the extensive and practical work undertaken by Professor Franz Ruppert, who worked alongside Hellinger many years ago and got to know him as a person. It may be found that working with a parent so that they come to see and feel what is of primary concern to them in their unique situation has the potential to heal and transform not only the individual but also the family dynamics and, in particular, a young offspring who otherwise might carry a disturbing legacy of unresolved trauma. Hence constellation work used in this way, rather than directly with a young child, may greatly assist the child through otherwise unresolved and disturbing difficulties. Further information can be found at www.franz-ruppert.de.

Primitive reflexes

Infant reflexes that do not integrate appropriately can cause symptoms such as an inability to concentrate or sit still, ADHD, sensory processing issues, co-ordination problems and learning disabilities, amongst other things. There are a number of approaches to working with retained primitive reflexes. These may involve exercises or touch to encourage primitive reflexes to be replaced by the more complex adult reflexes. Some of these were developed by Peter Blythe and are now taught by teachers trained at the Institute for Neuro-Physiological Psychology.

There are simple tests available that parents can do at home to see if some of the most common major reflexes are still active. These are available at www.retainedneonatalreflexes.com.au/test-at-hom.

Some of the more well-known primitive reflexes are:

- The Moro (or startle) reflex, which emerges at around nine weeks in utero and gets inhibited at anywhere between two and six months of life.

- The Asymmetrical Tonic Neck Reflex (ATNR), which emerges at around four months in utero and is inhibited at around five months after birth. This causes the arms to bend and the legs to extend when the head is in flexion, and the arms to extend and the legs to flex when the head is extended.

- The Spinal Galant, which emerges around the time of the Moro reflex but usually inhibits a little later.

- The sucking and rooting reflex, which starts at around four months in utero and inhibits at around four months after birth.

- The Babinski reflex, which starts at birth and inhibits anywhere up to two years of age.

Certain reflexes may be over-active, under-active or fail to inhibit. The Moro reflex, which involves the baby's arms going backwards, is a primitive startle reflex and is commonly seen. It involves a sudden strong activation of the sympathetic nervous system and a generally hyper-aroused state. In the second part of this reflex the parasympathetic system becomes more evident, with a closing of the arms over the chest. Babies who have had traumatic births can display this reflex just as they are dropping off to sleep, as though being off guard is perceived as dangerous. More information on primitive reflexes and how they affect child development can be found in the book *Reflexes, Learning and Behaviour: A Window into the Child's Mind* by Sally Goddard (Fern Ridge, 2005).

Rhythmic Movement Training

Rhythmic Movement Training (RMT) provides training and certification internationally and in the UK. It is open to anyone; often parents, teachers and various health practitioners find this a useful method of working 'one-to-one' with young children who may be experiencing various difficulties, many of which are outlined in this book. The training provides detailed information about child development and normal and 'trapped' reflexes, equipping those who attend with practical skills and help through movement, isometric pressure and gentle rocking exercises.

An RMT therapist may find that encouraging a parent to use these practical skills with their own child is also beneficial, given the need to work extremely sensitively and safely with babies and young children. Further information can be found at www.rhythmicmovement.co.uk.

EARLY TRAUMA INFORMATION

All of us have experienced some degree of stress or trauma in our early life. Some is medically necessary. The long-term impact is in proportion to the severity and length of the trauma, as well as the degree to which the trauma interferes with the child connecting with its mother and father. Any event is less traumatic if accompanied by loving support and connection.

Some known causes of early trauma

- Unwelcoming or fearful feelings at discovery of pregnancy

- Stressful or abusive relationship between parents during pregnancy or after birth

- Maternal stress, fear or depression during pregnancy or infancy

- Child was not wanted for some part of pregnancy

- Considered or attempted abortion

- Biochemical stresses during pregnancy from nicotine, alcohol, pesticides, and so on

- Twin lost during pregnancy, including early pregnancy or during birth

- Chemical induction of labour

- Foetal monitors that are screwed into the skull of the foetus

- Premature birth

- NICU experience with all accompanying medical interventions

- Unusually long or unusually fast labour

- Being stuck during labour

- Cord tightly wrapped around the neck

- Near-death experience or deprivation of oxygen

- Medical interventions such as C-section, forceps, vacuum extraction

- Anaesthesia which breaks the contact between mother and baby

- Separation from the mother after birth or for extended periods during infancy

- Painful medical interventions such as heal sticks, spinal taps

- Maternal postpartum depression or strong anxiety

- Being given up for adoption

- Death in the family

- Unresolved traumatic history in parents or ancestors, such as early abuse, loss of a parent, traumatic birth, or being given up for adoption

- Hospitalization or surgery as an infant, including circumcision

- Any particularly painful accident, injury or illness.

Some signs that babies exhibit after experiencing trauma

- Glossed-over eyes

- Cross-eyes or divergent eyes

- Total or partial inability to orient when confronted by new surroundings

- Too little tone or too much tension in their muscles

- Startle response to sound or movement

- Jerky arms, legs and head

- Involuntary shaking or tremors

- Constant, weak or 'absent' crying

- High-pitched crying sounds

- Inconsolable crying and crying without apparent cause

- Hypersensitivity to near or direct touch

- Desire to not be held

- Falling asleep when over-stimulated

- Inability to grasp

- Nursing/feeding difficulties

- Arching

- Splaying hands

- Excessive hiccups

- Frequent gagging

- Avoidance of eye contact.

Some signs that older children exhibit after experiencing trauma

- Hyperactivity

- Coordination and balance problems

- Gait problems

- Toilet training challenges

- Speech delays

- Learning disabilities

- Tantrums

- Inappropriate aggression/timidity

- Depression

- Nightmares

- Response out of proportion to stimulus

- Inability to make eye contact

- Inability to ask for help

- Rage toward parent(s) or others

- Hypersensitivity

- Health challenges such as asthma and seizures

- Harmful behaviour towards siblings

- Tactile defensiveness (desire to not be touched).

Common parental responses to a child's early trauma

When a baby or child is less available for bonding and attachment due to early trauma, the baby or child may not respond as expected to parental attempts to soothe, comfort and connect. This can affect the parents' responses. Some parental responses include:

- Overwhelm

- Shame/guilt

- Exhaustion

- Sleeplessness

- Anxiety

- Stress

- Helplessness

- Anger

- Frustration

- Postpartum depression or anxiety

- Numbness

- Conflict between parents

- Difficulty asking for support.

Common signs in adults of early trauma

All of us have experienced early stress or trauma to one degree or another. Unresolved early trauma can significantly interfere with current daily life. As more recent traumatic events occur, they layer on top of our earliest imprinting. In fact, our ability to recover from traumatic events as older children and adults is dependent on our resilience or lack of it due to our earliest traumatic imprinting. Teens and adults can manifest any of the signs listed under children, plus:

- Difficulty in forming and maintaining a healthy primary relationship with a partner

- Aggression manifested as acting out, destructive or criminal behaviour

- Excessive timidity in everyday life

- Inappropriate flight or fight response to non-threatening circumstances

- Difficulty mobilizing effectively in the face of real aggression or danger

- Difficulty in setting healthy limits and boundaries, saying 'no' when appropriate

- Merging inappropriately with others to one's own detriment

- Difficulty in responding empathetically to others

- Confusion, difficulty making decisions

- Self-destructive behaviours such as drug and alcohol abuse, physical mutilation, over- or under-eating

- Excessive risk-taking, dangerous driving, disregarding the safety of others

- Forced sex or having unprotected sex when children are not wanted

- Failing to take responsibility for one's actions, blaming others

- Difficulty setting appropriate goals and working towards them

- Difficulty in foreseeing the consequences of one's actions

- Consistent difficulty with some aspect of a task: intention, preparation, action, follow-through or integration

- Difficulty holding a job or establishing oneself in a satisfying career

- Inability to successfully establish oneself in the world as an independent adult

- Difficulties in parenting, abusive or neglectful behaviour towards children

- Difficulty in establishing an effective support system of family, friends, teachers, mentors and/or professionals.

Source

BEBA (2016) *About Early Trauma.* Santa Barbara, CA: BEBA. Available at http://beba.org/early-traum, accessed on 7 October 2016.

CHARACTERISTICS, BEHAVIOURS AND ABILITIES OF THE NON-TRAUMATIZED AND TRAUMATIZED NEONATE

Non-traumatized neonate demonstrate the following characteristics, abilities and behaviours

- Eyes are clear and present

- Eyes coordinate, normal convergence

- Ability to orient to visual, auditory and tactile stimuli

- Ability to smoothly move from one sensory stimuli to another without breaks in movement continuity

- General balanced tonicity throughout the body

- Appropriate homeostatic autonomic responses to stimuli (i.e. if the light changes, the pupils will respond in kind; if activity demands change, respiratory and pulse responses will meet the demand)

- Moro or startle response present with clear and present danger only

- Movements of the extremities smooth and without breaks in continuity

- Smooth trunk movements of the body in flexion, extension, lateral flexion and rotation movements at will

- Accurate proprioception (they know where they are in space)

- Strong sucking response

- Holds head up and turns head from side to side to orient at will

- Balanced cervical and sub-occipital muscle tone

- Absence of shaking or tremors

- Deliberate response to near or direct touch

- Matches gentle tactile pressure with extremities, head or trunk of body

- Crying corresponds to need

- Able to cry with full range of sounds and emotional content

- Able to differentiate emotional expressions

- Enjoys experimenting with movements, sounds and expressions

- Body positions and movement patterns do not interrupt ability to orient

- Vibrant skin colour

- Chooses to make contact deliberately

- Voluntarily moves attention from inside to outside

- Shows interest in new experience

- Voluntarily grasps

- Moves to mother's breast, latches on and feeds.

Subtle energetic, fluid tide and cranial characteristics of non-traumatized neonates

- Full palpable energy field with distinct clear boundaries

- Free flow of vital energy throughout the body

- Round, full cranium, absence of cranial moulding

- Full strong potency of vital fluid tides

- Full fluid tide inspiration and expiration patterns with appropriate physiologic reciprocity

- Easy expansion and contraction of the cranial field within normal physiologic movement patterns

- Able to meet stress with appropriate energetic fluid responses, lateral fluctuations, and still points.

Shock affect characteristics in neonates

- Glassy eyes

- Eyes do not converge normally, but cross or split

- Total or partial inability to orient to visual, auditory and tactile stimuli

- Generalized or body area specific hypertonicity

- Involuntary changes in autonomic responses including pulse, respiratory rate, skin colour changes, pupil changes in the eye

- Moro response or startle response to sound or movement

- Jerking movements of extremities

- Inability to hold head up

- Hypermobility of neck, especially at atlanto-occipital junction

- Involuntary shaking or tremors

- Tactile sensitivity to near or direct touch

- Total or partial inability to match gentle pressure from direct touch with extremities, head or trunk of body

- Weak, hollow or empty crying sounds

- High-pitched crying sounds

- Crying inconsolably, getting lost in their emotions without ability to make visual, auditory or tactile contact

- Frequent crying without apparent reason

- Lack of skin colour

- Total or partial absence of alertness during awake states

- Withdrawal sleep to light, sound or movement sensory stimulation

- Inability to voluntarily shuttle attention from inside to outside or outside to inside

- Inability to grasp.

Subtle energetic, fluid tide and cranial shock affect indicators

- Weak energy field without clear boundaries

- Erratic energy field patterns

- Counter-clockwise umbilical pattern

- Unresolved cranial moulding

- Unresolved postural patterns

- Weak potency within vital fluid tide

- Total or partial inability of fluid tide potency to build

- Long, weak still points

- Stops in the fluid tide patterns

- Cranial strain patterns

- Non-physiologic cranial movement pattern.

Source

Castellino, R. (1996) *Being with Newborns: An Introduction to Somatotropic Therapy; Attention to the Newborn; Healing Betrayal, New Hope for the Prevention of Violence.* Santa Barbara, CA: Castellino Training.

ACETAMINOPHEN (PARACETAMOL) AND AUTISM

Dr Carolyn Goh

The prevalence of autism in the USA and the UK has increased dramatically in the last 10 years but the jury is still out on a definite cause. Although a common time frame seems to be around vaccinations there are a growing number of parents who have not vaccinated their child and yet they are on the ASD spectrum.

The scientist Steve Schultz, in his quest to understand a cause for his son's autism, came up with an interesting hypothesis. In his book *Understanding Autism: My quest for Nathan* he writes: 'Then I remembered that Nathan had gotten so sick from the MMR vaccine and how I had given him so much acetaminophen. Perhaps there was something about acetaminophen'.

Acetaminophen is also termed paracetamol, is used to treat pain and fever, and has become one of the most popular over the counter non-narcotic analgesic agents. A large multinational study by Beasley *et al.* (2008) found a dose dependent association between use of acetaminophen and asthma, rhinoconjuctivitis, and eczema. A number of published papers describe the mechanisms by which acetaminophen can induce inflammation by altering toxin metabolism and inflammatory processes in the body (Becker and Schultz, 2010; Schultz 2010; Good 2009; Shaw 2013).

Bauer and Kriebel (2013) conducted an epidemiologic study suggesting that the use of acetaminophen at the time of circumcision might account for many cases of autism. The authors found that after acetaminophen became commonly used to treat circumcision pain after 1995, there was a strong correlation between country level (n = 9) autism/ASD prevalence in males and a country's circumcision rate (r = 0.98).

Schultz carried out a case-control study published in 2008 showing Acetaminophen use after measles-mumps-rubella vaccination was significantly associated with autistic disorder in children 5 years of age or less. Shaw (2013) reported that Cuba – with an autism incidence a fraction of the US (1/300th) requires vaccinations but prohibits over-the-counter acetaminophen, and only rarely gives acetaminophen before vaccinations.

What about the use of acetaminophen during pregnancy? In 2013, Bauer *et al.* reported that prenatal use of acetaminophen was strongly correlated with autism/ASD. This was further supported by studies from Brandlistuen (2013) and Liew (2014).

In his latest paper, Schultz (2016) recommends that acetaminophen use be reviewed for safety in children. Calpol and Tylenol (US) are still the 'go to' remedy to soothe teething toddlers and reduce fevers. As the research unfolds, it is best to err on the side of caution and choose medications that do not contain acetaminophen. It is also a good idea to check medicines before they are given to your child by a health practitioner.

References

Posadas I, Santos P, Blanco A, Muñoz-Fernández M, Ceña V. Acetaminophen induces apoptosis in rat cortical neurons. PLoS ONE. 2010;15(12):e15360.

Beasley, R., Clayton T, Crane J, von Mutius E, Lai CK, Montefort S, Stewart A ., Association between paracetamol use in infancy and childhood, and risk of asthma, rhinoconjunctivitis, and eczema in children aged 6-7 years: analysis from Phase Three of the ISAAC programme. Lancet, 2008. 372(9643): p. 1039-48.

Becker, K.G. and S.T. Schultz, Similarities in features of autism and asthma and a possible link to acetaminophen use. Medical Hypotheses, 2010. 74(1): p. 7-11.

Schultz, S.T., Can autism be triggered by acetaminophen activation of the endocannabinoid system? Acta Neurobiologiae Experimentalis (Warsaw), 2010. 70(2): p. 227-231.

Good, P., Did acetaminophen provoke the autism epidemic? Alternative Medicine Review, 2009. 14(4): p. 364-372.

Shaw, W., Evidence that Increased Acetaminophen use in Genetically Vulnerable Children Appears to be a Major Cause of the Epidemics of Autism, Attention Deficit with Hyperactivity, and Asthma. Journal of Restorative Medicine, 2013. 2: p. 1-16.

Bauer, A. and D. Kriebel, Prenatal and perinatal analgesic exposure and autism: an ecological link. Environmental Health, 2013. 12(1): p. 41.

Schultz ST, Klonoff-Cohen HS, Wingard DL, Akshoomoff NA, Macera CA, Ji M. Acetaminophen (paracetamol) use, measles-mumps-rubella vaccination, and autistic disorder: the results of a parent survey. Autism 2008;12(3): 293–307.

Brandlistuen, R.E., Ystrom E., Nulman I., Koren. G., Nordeng. H., Prenatal paracetamol exposure and child neurodevelopment: a sibling-controlled cohort study. International Journal of Epidemiology, 2013. 42(6): p. 1702-1713.

Liew, Z., Ritz B, Rebordosa C, Lee PC, Olsen J, Acetaminophen use during pregnancy, behavioral problems, and hyperkinetic disorders. JAMA Pediatr, 2014. 168(4): p. 313-20.

Schultz ST. & Gould GG. Acetaminophen Use for Fever in Children Associated with Autism Spectrum Disorder. Autism Open Access. 2016 Apr;6(2). pii: 170.

RESOURCES

This section provides a list of organizations providing access to training or to databases of therapists working with babies and children. This list is by no means exhaustive and does not imply endorsement by the authors or publishers.

Pre- and perinatal psychology associations and teaching organizations

Association for Prenatal and Perinatal Psychology and Health

> https://birthpsychology.com

The International Society for Prenatal and Perinatal Psychology and Medicine

> www.isppm.de

Institute of Pre- and Perinatal Education (Karlton Terry)

> www.IPPE.info

Conscious Embodiment Trainings

> www.conscious-embodiment.co.uk

Enhancing the Future

> www.enhancingthefuture.co.uk

BEBA

> http://beba.org

First Expression (David Haas)

    www.first-expression.co.uk

Ray Castellino

    www.castellinotraining.com

    http://raycastellino.com/referrals/graduates.php

William Emerson

    http://emersonbirthrx.com

Thomas Harms

    http://thomasharms.org

Ehealth Learning

    www.ehealthlearning.tv

Schools and teaching organizations of manual therapies working with babies and children
Osteopathy and Cranial Osteopathy

    www.osteopathy.org

    www.bcom.ac.uk/students/postgraduate/pgcert-childrens-osteopathy

Sutherland Cranial College

    www.scco.ac

Craniosacral Therapy
Karuna Institute

    www.karuna-institute.co.uk

Craniosacral Therapy Educational Trust (CTET)

    www.cranio.co.uk

College of Cranio-Sacral Therapy

www.ccst.co.uk

Upledger Institute

www.upledger.com

Bowen Technique

Bowen Therapy Academy of Australia

www.bowtech.com

Bowen Training UK

www.bowentraining.co.uk

Bowen Therapy Academy of Europe

www.bowtech.at

John Wilks

www.therapy-training.com

Baby massage

International Association of Infant Massage

www.iaim.org.uk

Childways

www.childways.co.uk

London School of Massage

www.londonschoolofmassage.co.uk

Play Therapy

http://playtherapy.org.uk

Filial Therapy

www.filialtherapy.co.uk

Equine Assisted Therapy

LEAP

www.leapequine.com

Children's Foundation for Equine Assisted Therapy

www.childrensfeat.org

Equine Assisted Psychotherapy and Learning

www.eagala.org

Stable Relationships

www.stable-relationships.com

Equine Facilitated Human Development

www.ifeal.me

Dyadic Developmental Psychotherapy

http://ddpnetwork.org

Infant Physical Therapy

www.birthinjuryguide.org

Theraplay

www.theraplay.org

Constellations Therapy

Centre for Systemic Constellations

  www.thecsc.net

Contact details for practitioners, clinics and other organizations specializing in treating babies and children

Bowen Technique

Bowen Association UK

  www.bowen-technique.co.uk

Bowen USA

  www.americanbowen.academy

Bowen Children's Clinics

  www.bowentherapy.org.uk

Craniosacral Therapy

Craniosacral Therapy Association of the UK

  www.craniosacral.co.uk

Biodynamic Craniosacral Therapy Association of North America

  www.craniosacraltherapy.org

Osteopathy

Osteopathic Centre for Children

  http://occ.uk.com

British School of Osteopathy clinics for babies and children

  www.bso.ac.uk/information-for-patients/specialist-and-community-clinics/#babiesandchildren

Child psychologists

www.achippp.org.uk/directory

Primitive reflexes

Institute of Neuro-Physiological Psychology (INPP)

www.inpp.org.uk

INPP USA

http://inpptrainingusa.com

Sound Learning Centre

www.thesoundlearningcentre.co.uk

Crossroads Institute

www.crossroadsinstitute.org

New Zealand

www.smartlearning.co.nz

David Mulhall

www.davidmulhall.co.uk

AUTHOR BIOGRAPHIES

Editor

John Wilks is the author of four books on complementary therapies and a contributing author to a recent book on Hypermobility Syndromes. His book *Choices in Pregnancy and Childbirth* was published by Singing Dragon in 2015 and has received much critical acclaim. He has been practising the Bowen Technique and Craniosacral Therapy since 1995, and works at three clinics in the south west of England. He has taught workshops on working with babies and mothers in many countries throughout the world including the UK, USA, South Africa, Germany, Denmark, Portugal, Norway, Bulgaria, Israel, Australia, Austria and France. In 2005 he set up a two-year practitioner training for midwives in Craniosacral Therapy, the first of its kind to be accredited by the Royal College of Midwives, and runs a large online training school for therapists at *www.ehealthlearning.tv* and *www.cyma.org.uk*.

Contributing authors

Matthew Appleton co-founded Conscious Embodiment Trainings with his partner Jenni Meyer, and is a registered craniosacral therapist and psychotherapist working in Bristol. He trained in Body Psychotherapy at the Wilhelm Reich Institute of Integrated Therapy in Germany and in Core Process Psychotherapy at the Karuna Institute in Devon. He further trained and assisted with the Institute of Pre- and Perinatal Education and is a member of the International Society of Prenatal and Perinatal Psychology and Medicine. For ten years he worked as a houseparent at A.S. Neill's famous democratic school Summerhill. His book A Free Range Childhood based on his experiences at Summerhill has been published in several languages. He developed and began teaching Integrative Baby Therapy (IBT) in 2010. Along with facilitating experiential workshops for adults, the main focus of his work is training practitioners in IBT in several European countries. *www.conscious-embodiment.co.uk*

Dr Carolyn Goh is a medically qualified doctor as well as holding a Bachelors in Engineering, a Masters in Bioengineering and a PhD in Bioengineering. Whilst completing her PhD at Imperial College London in the Analysis of Infants' Heart Rate Signals and Sudden Infant Death Syndrome, she discovered the Bowen Technique and was struck by its healing potential. She currently runs a private Bowen Therapy practice from Violet Hill Studios in St Johns Wood, London. She is author of the following self-help e-books: *Baby Bowen – Natural Colic Relief; Stop Wheezing, Start Breathing – The Bowen Technique for Asthma* (with Alastair Rattray); and *Bowen for Pregnancy and Labour – A Self Help Guide to Relieving Your Aches and Pains in Pregnancy.* She was a contributing author to *Using the Bowen Technique* and *Choices in Pregnancy and Childbirth* published by Singing Dragon. *http://bowentechniquelondon.co.uk*

David Haas originally graduated as a chartered electrical engineer in the 1970s and has been a complementary therapist since the early 1990s. Within his engineering degree, one area of study was the theory of electric fields. It was during his training as a polarity therapist that he became aware of the energy field systems of the human body and how they may also be involved in the way we connect with others. Within his polarity therapy studies he developed an interest in early life and began to realize the possibilities of how supporting babies and their families could make a difference in these very early relationships; how that could have an effect, not just within that family, but also in the different forms of relationship within society. He studied Craniosacral Therapy with Franklyn Sills at the Karuna Institute in Devon and Pre- and Perinatal Therapy with Ray Castellino, initially in Devon and then in California. He has assisted Ray on several trainings and is a certified Womb Surround Process Workshop facilitator and a supervisor in this work. David is a registered craniosacral therapist and craniosacral therapy supervisor. He founded First Expression as a container for working and training within this early life period. He teaches seminars and runs workshops in the UK and internationally. David practises at a multidisciplinary clinic in Surrey and in London. He is currently training as a Somatic Experiencing Practitioner (SEP). *www.first-expression.co.uk*

Thomas Harms lives and works in Bremen, Germany, and has been working in the field of body psychotherapy for over 25 years with adults, couples and infants. He founded, with his wife Karin Meyer-Harms, an outpatient clinic, the Centre for Primary Prevention and Body Psychotherapy (ZePP), and in 1993 the Crybaby Clinic in Berlin. This was first cry outpatient clinic for parents with excessively crying babies. From this work he developed his approach which he terms 'Emotional First Aid', which is a body-psychotherapeutic model of acute intervention that he teaches in Germany and across Europe. His main focus is on working with regulatory and attachment dysfunction in the first year of life caused by trauma and also working with adults with traumatic early attachment and developmental experiences. *www.thomasharms.org*

Anita Hegerty studied Cellular Pathology at Bristol and completed her PhD thesis five years later. She graduated from the British School of Osteopathy in 1990 and was involved in the Children's Clinic and the Expectant Mothers' Clinic there. Since qualifying as an osteopath she has completed two extended residential postgraduate courses in Osteopathy in the Cranial Field. She is currently enrolled onto the Advanced Diploma in Paediatric Osteopathy run by the SCCO (Sutherland Cranial College of Osteopathy) and also trained as a Developmental Baby Massage Teacher. She was a contributing author to *Choices in Pregnancy and Childbirth*. *www.glencairnhouse.co.uk*

Graham Kennedy has been a therapist for over 20 years, specializing in working with attachment and early life trauma. He is a teacher and practitioner of Craniosacral Therapy, and was the co-founder and joint principal of the Institute of Craniosacral Studies. He also has a background in prenatal and birth psychology, and has taught trainings in the UK, Italy, Germany and South Africa. Graham is also a trainer and parent consultant for Adoption UK, the largest adoption support charity in the UK. He is currently training as an Integrative Child Psychotherapist. *www.enhancingthefuture.co.uk*

Kate Rosati, RCST, RM, IBCLC, is a registered craniosacral therapist, midwife and lactation consultant living and working in Alton, Hampshire, UK. She trained as a craniosacral therapist in 2007 and since then has assisted on many courses with Graham Kennedy, Matthew Appleton and Conscious Embodiment Trainings.

Professor Franz Ruppert is Professor of Psychology at the University of Applied Sciences in Munich, a post he has held since 1992. Since 1995 he has focused on psychotherapeutic work and specifically on the causes of psychosis, schizophrenia and other forms of severe mental illness. He has combined with this his interest in bonding and attachment theories and modern trauma work in order to better understand the effect of traumatic events, not just for those who suffer the event, but on whole bonding systems such as families. He came into contact with the Systemic constellations work of Bert Hellinger in Germany in the mid-1990s and since then has utilized this methodology in order to work with clients and understand the subtle and hidden dynamics of trauma in systems. He teaches trauma theory at the University of Applied Sciences, works with individuals and facilitates workshops in Germany and many other countries, including the UK. *www.franz-ruppert.de*

Michael Shea, PhD, is one of the pre-eminent educators and authors in the fields of somatic psychology, myofascial release and Craniosacral Therapy. He presents seminars throughout the US, Canada and Europe. He received his master's degree in Buddhist Psychology at Naropa University, and a doctorate in Somatic Psychology at The Union Institute. Dr Shea was certified in 1986 as one of the first Full Instructors of CranioSacral Therapy by the Upledger Institute and was an advanced Rolfer for 20 years. He is currently adjunct faculty and teaches human embryology in the pre- and perinatal psychology doctoral programmes at the Santa Barbara Graduate Institute in California. His clinical focus is on treating infants and children with neurological problems and developmental delays. This also includes teaching clinical skills for adults that carry pre- and perinatal trauma. Dr Shea is the author of a number of books, including *Somatic Psychology* and *Biodynamic Craniosacral Therapy – Volume 1 and Volume 2*. He has been a Florida Licensed Massage Therapist since 1976. He is a founding member of the International Affiliation of Biodynamic Trainings and the Massage Therapy Body of Knowledge task force (MTBOK). He makes his home in South Florida with his wife, Cathy. *www.michaelsheateaching.com*

Ann Diamond Weinstein, PhD, is a Preconception, Prenatal and Early Parenting Specialist with a doctorate in Prenatal and Perinatal Psychology. In her consultation practice in the USA she provides education and coaching to individuals, families, professionals and groups on issues related to preconception, pregnancy, birth and early parenting experiences, and their impacts over the lifespan. Ann Diamond Weinstein's work with women and families spans three decades. The origins of her current work as a Preconception, Prenatal and Early Parenting Specialist began with her work as a Certified Childbirth Educator for 13 years, and later a Birth Doula. During this time she provided education and support to women and their families through their experiences of pregnancy, birth and the early postnatal period. As an educator and coach Dr Weinstein focuses on stress management and issues relating to preconception, pregnancy, birth and early parenting experiences. Her recent book *Prenatal Development and Parents' Lived Experiences – How Early Events Shape Our Psychophysiology and Relationships* was published in 2016 as part of the Norton series on Interpersonal Neurobiology. *http://anndiamondweinstein.com*

SUBJECT INDEX

AUTHOR INDEX